Physiological Principles in Medicine

General Editors

Dr. R.N. Hardy
Physiological Laboratory, Cambridge

Professor M. Hobsley
Department of Surgical Studies, The Middlesex Hospital and The
Middlesex Hospital Medical School, London

Professor K.B. Saunders
Department of Medicine, St George's Hospital and St George's Hospital
Medical School, London

Dr. J.T. Fitzsimons
Physiological Laboratory, Cambridge

Physiological Principles in Medicine

Books are published in linked pairs—the preclinical volume linked to its clinical counterpart as follows:

Endocrine Physiology by Richard N. Hardy
Clinical Endocrinology by Peter Daggett

Digestive System Physiology by Paul A. Sanford
Disorders of the Digestive System by Michael Hobsley

Respiratory Physiology by John Widdicombe and Andrew Davies
Respiratory Disorders by Ian Cameron and Nigel T. Bateman

Neurophysiology by R.H.S. Carpenter

Reproduction and the Fetus by Alan L.R. Findlay
Gynaecology, Obstetrics and the Neonate by S.J. Steele

In preparation:

Clinical Neurology by C.D. Marsden

Gynaecology, Obstetrics and the Neonate

S.J. Steele

Director, The Academic Department of Obstetrics and Gynaecology,
The Middlesex Hospital London

with a contribution (Chapters 3, 4 and 5, and 8 jointly) by
N.R.C. Roberton
Consultant Paediatrician, Cambridge Maternity Hospital;
Associate Lecturer in Paediatrics, Cambridge University;
Fellow of Fitzwilliam College, Cambridge.

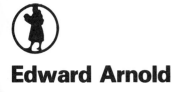

Edward Arnold

© S.J. Steele 1985

First published 1985
by Edward Arnold (Publishers) Ltd
41 Bedford Square
London WC1B 3DQ

Edward Arnold (Australia) Pty Ltd
80 Waverly Road
Caulfield East 3145
PO Box 234
Melbourne

Edward Arnold
300 North Charles Street
Baltimore
Maryland 21201

British Library Cataloguing in Publication Data

Steele, S.J.
  Gynaecology, obstetrics and the neonate.—
  (Physiological principles in medicine, ISSN
  0260-2946)
  1. Gynecology   2. Obstetrics
  I. Title   II. Series
  618   RG101

  ISBN 0-7131-4455-6

Filmset in 10/11pt Baskerville by
CK Typesetters Ltd, 26 Mulgrave Road, Sutton, Surrey
Printed and Bound in Great Britain by Thomson Litho Ltd, East Kilbride

General preface to series

Student textbooks of medicine seek to present the subject of human diseases and their treatment in a manner that is not only informative, but interesting and readily assimilable. It is important, in a field where knowledge advances rapidly, that principles are emphasized rather than details, so that what is contained in the book remains valid for as long as possible.

These considerations favour an approach which concentrates on each disease as a disturbance of normal structure and function. Rational therapy follows logically from a knowledge of the disturbance, and it is in this field where some of the most rapid advances in Medicine have occurred.

A disturbance of normal structure without any disturbance of function may not be important to the patient except for cosmetic or psychological reasons. Therefore, it is disturbances in function that should be stressed. Preclinical students should aim at a comprehensive understanding of physiological principles so that when they arrive on the wards they will be able to appreciate the significance of disordered function in disease. Clinical students must be presented with descriptions of disease which stress the disturbances in normal physiological functions that are responsible for the symptoms and signs which they find in their patients. All students must be made aware of the growing points in physiology which, even though not immediately applicable to the practice of Medicine, will almost certainly become so during the course of their professional lives.

In this Series, the major physiological systems are each covered by a pair of books, one preclinical and the other clinical, in which the authors have attempted to meet the requirements discussed above. A particular feature is the provision of numerous cross-references between the two members of a pair of books to facilitate the blending of basic science and clinical expertise that is the goal of this Series. This coordination, which is initiated at the planning stage and continues throughout the writing of each pair of books, is achieved by frequent discussions between the preclinical and clinical authors concerned and between them and the editors of the Series.

RNH   KBS
MH   JTF

Preface

Gynaecology, Obstetrics and the Neonate is intended to meet the need of medical and other students, and doctors preparing for diplomas in obstetrics and gynaecology. It is hoped also that students who have become familiar with its contents, will find it useful for reference once they have qualified. Detailed descriptions of practical procedures, notably normal delivery, are not included since every student should have ample opportunity to see, learn and practice these techniques during the part of their course devoted to obstetrics and gynaecology. In contrast to other disciplines most patients are not ill and students should adjust their attitudes and treatment appropriately as well as acquiring the necessary skills.

In gynaecology the problems range from carcinoma to sexual difficulties, and preventative aspects include screening for malignant disease and contraception. Obstetrics involves the conditions which threaten the mother's life, technical difficulties sometimes associated with delivery, and the possible disasters of the birth of an abnormal baby or perinatal death. In no area of medicine is it more important to be able to listen to the patient, to be sensitive to her need for help and probable embarrassment and to conduct examinations with appropriate privacy and gentleness. As a gynaecologist one meets patients of all ages and the specialty comprises a blend of medicine, endocrinology, surgery and psychology. I hope that readers of this book will find their clinical work as fascinating and rewarding as I have. The doctor who uses common sense in applying basic knowledge of obstetrics and gynaecology is usually safe and with this in mind I have presented much of the material in relation to problems, but the onus is on the doctor to identify these correctly.

It is sad that Dick Hardy did not live to see this volume published and I must record my appreciation of his early encouragement. I am also particularly grateful to Alan Findlay and Cliff Roberton, my paediatric co-author, with whom it has been a pleasure to work. I must also record my gratitude to John Guillebaud for advice on Chapter 15, Judy Adams for the ultrasound pictures, Paul Price for support and patience and to Pratibha Kothari and Jeannie Sloman for invaluable secretarial assistance.

London, 1984   S.J. Steele

Contents of Findlay, Reproduction and the Fetus

While reading this book you will find it helpful to refer to the companion volume *Reproduction and the Fetus* by Alan L.R. Findlay.

Contents

1

Normal pregnancy

Diagnosis

The commonest reason for suspecting pregnancy is the failure to menstruate at the expected time.* This prompts many women to seek medical advice or obtain a pregnancy test though other symptoms may, by their presence or absence, make the diagnosis more or less likely. Anyone who has been pregnant before will be likely to recognize the symptoms. Women who do not wish to be pregnant may not seek advice, ignoring the possibility of pregnancy. Those with irregular cycles, and any who suffer bleeding early in pregnancy may not recognize the possibility and so may present at a more advanced stage of pregnancy than others.

In addition to amenorrhoea (absence of periods) the symptoms of early pregnancy are:

1. Discomfort and enlargement of breasts.
2. Frequency of micturition (diurnal and nocturnal).
3. Gastro-intestinal symptoms: altered appetite (quantity and preferences), nausea and vomiting, abdominal discomfort, constipation.
4. Tiredness and some change in mood.

These symptoms are all common but they do not occur in every pregnancy and when they do they vary greatly in degree. If a patient seeks advice as to whether she is pregnant many doctors first do a pregnancy test. In fact, the history will often indicate whether pregnancy is likely and this should be complemented by examination. The signs of pregnancy are:

1. Breast changes. Increased vascularity, obvious enlargement and tenderness occur first; pigmentation of the areola and enlargement of Montgomery's tubercles follow, with the production of colostrum which may be expressed by the fifth month (some secretion is normal in women previously pregnant and this test should only be attempted gently — rough or vigorous attempts can be very painful).

2. Enlargement of the uterus; the most important sign, detectable often by an experienced obstetrician at 6 weeks. After 12 weeks the uterus is usually palpable above the pubis.

---

*For relevant physiology see Findlay *Reproduction and the Fetus*, Chapter 6.

3. Softening of the uterus which is variable and may make it difficult to feel or easily mistaken for a cyst.

4. Increased vascularity of the cervix and vagina leads in some cases to a blue appearance (compared with the normal pink) and increased secretion and warmth.

Pregnancy tests

These are based on the detection of (human) Chorionic Gonadotrophin (hCG) in urine by immunological means. They are best used on early morning specimens of urine which are positive approximately 3 weeks after conception (5 weeks after the start of the last period when the cycle is regular). However, there is some variation in the reliability of the tests and in most women's menstrual cycles, so that it is often best to seek a test 40 or more days after the first day of the last period if the cycle is approximately 28 days and regular. Women with cycles of 35 days or more will need to wait longer if a pregnancy test is to be of value. In advanced pregnancy, because hCG levels start to fall after 12 weeks, these tests may be falsely negative, particularly in the second half of pregnancy, and this is one good reason why patients should be examined before having a pregnancy test. High levels of LH can produce a false positive test.

Assays of the β subunit of chorionic gonadotrophin are now available in some places and these can detect pregnancy before the period is missed. Another useful aid to the diagnosis of early pregnancy is ultrasound, which can detect the gestation sac and then the embryo. This is a very positive method since there can be no doubt once the embryo has been seen and this is normally possible at 6–7 weeks.

Once it is established that the woman is pregnant she should discuss with her doctor where she is going to have the baby and what arrangements need to be made. She or her doctor can then arrange for her to be seen at the appropriate antenatal clinic reasonably soon. It is desirable that patients be seen in the first trimester because this facilitates the early identification of possible problems and accurate dating of the pregnancy, while ensuring support for the woman if she suffers any complications. Those women with medical disorders, previous subfertility or obstetric complications or social problems particularly need early advice. Any who wish to have a termination should be counselled or referred for this within a short interval.

Antenatal care

This may be given by general practitioners, specialist obstetricians or both (shared care). Midwives are specially trained in obstetrics and can undertake much of the antenatal and postnatal care, as well as normal labour and delivery. Others such as health visitors, physiotherapists and social workers can also contribute.

A crucial decision is where the woman is to have her baby. She is entitled to ask for delivery where she wishes, subject to there being vacancies, but it is the duty of the doctors and midwives to advise her so that she makes a sensible decision. The facilities available in different units vary as do attitudes and these plus previous experience, if any, in particular hospitals, the distance from home, the local reputation of a unit as well as professional advice contribute to the final decision. If there is an above average risk of a complication the doctor has a duty to press the woman strongly to go to a unit with full facilities. General practitioner units are designed to cope only with straightforward labours and deliveries, if problems arise or seem likely during pregnancy or labour the patient is normally transferred to a consultant unit. Close liaison between general practitioners and the staff of hospital consultant units facilitates this and in case of doubt the consultant can be asked for his opinion.

There is at present pressure for women to have greater opportunities to deliver at home; this represents a swing of the pendulum since the time some years ago, when a significant number of babies were delivered at home and there was strong demand for everyone to be able to have their babies in hospital. It represents also some dissatisfaction with the conveyor belt attitudes and regimes, and poor communication in some units. There are some emergencies and complications which can occur unexpectedly in labour or delivery; inevitably therefore delivery at home must be more hazardous than in hospital and for this reason most obstetricians advise against home delivery. At the same time the preference of many women for confinement in homely surroundings with husband and perhaps children present is understandable and laudable. As a result of this demand some less clinical delivery (birthing) rooms are being provided. There is considerable choice in the arrangements for hospital confinement ranging from a 10 days stay after delivery, to a 48 hour stay or return home within a few hours of delivery (called the domino system), these of course being elastic so that the stay can be lengthened or treatment altered if necessary. Another desire among women is for continuity of care and for familiar staff, particularly midwives, to look after them at delivery.

Many women are frightened of hospitals and the professionals involved in obstetric care, and there is a need to improve their confidence by better education and communication, as well as by more sympathetic and considerate treatment. There are physiological grounds for believing that the confident relaxed mother will have a better labour than one who is apprehensive.

Objectives of antenatal care:

To enable the woman to have her baby as safely, normally and happily as possible.

To ensure that the baby is born alive and as healthy as possible.

To identify any medical disorder particularly if it is likely to affect pregnancy

To educate a woman to keep as fit as possible during the pregnancy and after it.

To prepare for the stress and discomfort of labour and for the subsequent care of her infant.

To support her in such a way that she can cope with the anxieties and problems of pregnancy, as well as her other responsibilities.

This may involve the husband and other children, since the husband can contribute to the welfare and relaxation of his wife, while he and his children may suffer if the wife has to spend extra time in hospital or if anything goes amiss. Pregnancy and labour can end in disaster be it maternal death, stillbirth or the delivery of an abnormal child; though rare, it is important to remember this even though better health and good obstetric care render it a relatively small risk (see Chapter 8).

The booking clinic

Ideally the woman should attend this clinic when she is 8–12 weeks pregnant. A history is taken, a general and obstetric examination performed, investigations, treatment and future care organized, and the relevant forms or certificates filled in. The opportunity should be taken to give the patient as much information as soon as possible, to put her at her ease, and to give her confidence in herself and the professionals.

History
This comprises
1. General medical history.
2. Family history (with particular attention to diabetes and diseases which may be inherited).
3. Previous obstetric history, including details of the present health of the children.
4. The first day of the last menstrual period (check whether it was a normal period).
5. The usual menstrual cycle (including any variation).
6. Details of any drugs taken shortly before, or after conception (including the contraceptive pill).
7. The average consumption of alcohol and cigarettes.
8. The time taken to conceive and details of any investigation or treatment for infertility.
9. A social history.

Examination
The height, weight and blood pressure are recorded. A general medical examination with particular reference to the cardio-vascular system, respiratory system, the abdomen (scars of operations omitted from the history may be seen) and varicose veins is performed. Any other examination indicated by the history must, of course be carried out.

The breasts are inspected to anticipate any feeding problems, for example due to inverted or small nipples, and palpated as a screening procedure to exclude any tumour.

The abdomen is palpated to determine the height of the fundus and the size, shape and consistency of the uterus if it is palpable. When patients book late the fetal size, lie, presenting part, position and attitude (for defintion see p. 16) may be felt and the fetal heart heard or fetal movements felt.

Vaginal examination is performed early in pregnancy:

1. To confirm that the uterus is enlarged appropriately (i.e. to confirm pregnancy).

2. To establish as accurately as possible the size of the uterus (to estimate the duration of pregnancy).

3. To exclude abnormalities such as ovarian cysts, fibroids and gross abnormalities of the pelvis.

It is important that this is done but many women are particularly apprehensive about it and some fear it will cause a miscarriage. A gentle examination will do no harm and is much less traumatic than intercourse. The patient should be reassured appropriately but if she is very tense and frightened it may be wise to omit it. It is her decision whether to have one or not. This is a good opportunity to take a cervical smear.

Investigations
1. Cervical smear.
2. Vaginal swab if there is any pruritus or abnormal discharge.
3. Haemoglobin estimation.
4. ABO and rhesus grouping (antibodies if Rh negative).
5. Rubella antibody titre (to determine immunity or susceptibility).
6. Serological tests for syphilis (these vary in different units).
7. Midstream urine for culture.
8. Haemoglobin electrophoresis for those at risk of sickle cell disease or thalassaemia.
9. Australia antigen antibody titre for those from high risk areas or with a history of jaundice.
10. Ultrasound scan to determine maturity, exclude multiple pregnancy and look for congenital abnormalities.
11. Other investigations may be appropriate for particular patients.

Administration
The patient will need to be given details of the organization of the clinics she will attend, the arrangements for antenatal classes and the place of confinement. She is often given literature about the clinic and hospital, national insurance entitlements and pregnancy in general. Liaison with the general practitioner, midwife and any other professionals who are, or should be, involved is also important.

Specific advice and education
Patients usually have many questions to ask and it is important that as many as possible of these are answered, for example, the reason for investigations and their implications need to be explained. Each patient will have her own problems and this is the time to sort them out. There is an increasing tendency for husbands to come to clinics with their wives and when they do, they should be involved in the booking and the discussions that follow.

Smoking   in pregnancy is harmful. It is associated with increased perinatal mortality, lower birth weight, more abortions and diminished intelligence of the children. Those who smoke should be urged strongly to stop as there is benefit from this even part way through the pregnancy.

Alcohol can lead to the fetal alcohol syndrome which may include growth deficiency, characteristic facies, abnormalities of the central nervous system, cardiac and renal defects. The dangers of genuine alcoholism in pregnancy are obviously great and there is increasing evidence that alcohol is better avoided altogether.

Diet should include plenty of protein, fruit and vegetables and at least a pint of milk a day. Carbohydrates should be limited in those who start overweight. Obese patients should be encouraged to get detailed advice from the dietician early in pregnancy. There is some evidence that the diet at conception may affect the risk of fetal abnormality, particularly spina bifida, and it is desirable that women should be eating a good diet before and throughout pregnancy. It is usual to give iron and folic acid supplements to women; a good time to start is about 16 weeks, when most women have stopped feeling sick. Asian women should have vitamin D supplements.

Work In general women should stop work at about week 28 of pregnancy when they are eligible for the Maternity Allowance (paid weekly for 18 weeks) as most begin to find work onerous. Those with threatened abortions, multiple pregnancy, bad obstetric histories, medical problems or who find their work too tiring will need to stop or reduce their hours earlier. The legislation about the right to return to work is complicated. In the UK the pregnant woman is entitled to return to her job after pregnancy provided she has been in continuous employment for 2 years and stops at 28 weeks; she should, however, read the appropriate Government leaflet and discuss the position with her employers. The Allowance is dependent on the woman having paid National Insurance Contributions in the previous year. There is also a lump sum, the Maternity Grant, paid for each baby born subject to the woman or her husband having paid contributions in the previous year.

Education and preparation for labour and parenthood

Women having their first child often know very little about pregnancy and there is not time in the clinics to go through all that is necessary, though it is important that there is opportunity and time for questions and discussions with midwives and doctors. Normally there will be antenatal classes at which women, and often their husbands, can learn about pregnancy, labour and methods of relaxing. There are a number of specific methods of doing this and classes may be organized in hospital, at a midwives' clinic or by some other organization such as the National Childbirth Trust. It is important that women do not have their expectations raised unrealistically in relation to relief of pain and normal labour, since if this does happen and they experience a complication they tend to feel guilty or inadequate or to look, often unjustifiably, for a scapegoat. Films of labour may be helpful while meetings with labour ward staff and a tour of the unit help to lessen the fear of the unknown.

Mothercraft classes are also held to help the future mother prepare for the baby and the responsibility of caring for it. Contact with the health visitor who will help and advise about the feeding, care and developmental assessment of the infant is helpful, and it is customary for the health visitor to call on the mother during her pregnancy. If the confinement is to be at home, or there is to be an early discharge, the district midwife will call to see that facilities are adequate and the mother appropriately prepared.

Travel

It is obviously unwise to travel too far afield towards the end of pregnancy and air lines are strict about not carrying women within 6 weeks of the expected date of delivery. Those with a bad obstetric history or complications of any sort may also be advised not to travel far at least in the first trimester. In giving advice it is important to consider the effect of the journey, the area to be visited and the facilities available for care if an emergency should arise. Long journeys in small cars are particularly uncomfortable and couples should be advised to stop frequently (at least every 100 miles). In some places immunization against disease is required and specialist advice should be obtained about the use of vaccines, in general the greatest caution should be exercised with live vaccines. Those prone to travel sickness may be particularly badly affected during pregnancy.

Sexual activity

Orgasm is associated with contraction of the uterus but there is no reason to advise abstinence unless there is a bad obstetric history or a record of threatened abortion. As the uterus rises up in the abdomen it is wise for the woman not to have the man on top of her and sexual play and intercourse should be consciously gentle. Towards the end of pregnancy some doctors advise against sexual activity but in normal pregnancy there is probably little risk and couples should follow their own inclinations. The libido of many women alters during pregnancy and some may decide or prefer to abstain.

Other activities

Common sense will indicate the answer to most questions. Extra rest is essential, particularly for those who are working full time, and in the last 8 weeks all pregnant women should be urged to lie down for an hour and a half in the afternoon. Physical actitivies, sports, dancing, swimming and others can be continued, but the changes of pregnancy will quickly affect performance, balance and the energy required so that they should be carried on with discretion. Pregnancy is certainly not the time to start unfamiliar physical activities.

Drugs

It is difficult to determine whether a drug causes abnormality or not. The best advice is not to take any drug unless there is a very good reason for doing so, in which case there is often little option. The most dangerous time is the first trimester when women do not always realize they are pregnant. If a woman is worried after taking a preparation inadvertently she can be reassured that it is most unlikely to have caused harm; no doctor can say more than this and no one can say the baby will be normal because there is a 2 per cent risk of major abnormality in any pregnancy.

Drugs likely to affect the fetus adversely include:

1. Anticonvulsants.
2. Antithyroid drugs (Carbimazole, etc).
3. Chloramphenicol (Grey baby syndrome).
4. Corticosteroids appear to be associated with a small increase in the risk of cleft palate.
5. Diazepam is slowly metabolized and if given shortly before labour will depress the neonate. (All hypnotics and CNS depressants will affect the fetus.)
6. Insulin may cause neonatal hypoglycaemia.
7. Norethisterone can cause masculinization of a female fetus.
8. Stilboestrol can cause vaginal adenosis and carcinoma in female offspring.
9. Sulphonamides interfere with bile conjugation in the neonate and so can cause kernicterus.
10. Tetracycline stains developing teeth and bone.
11. Warfarin obviously predisposes to haemorrhage but can also produce chondrodysplasia punctata.

X-rays

Should be avoided in pregnancy unless there is a strong indication; as few films as possible should be taken, preferably avoiding the first trimester. The dangers are leukaemia or other neoplastic disease in the child and genetic damage to maternal or fetal gonads, though the risk is small.

Antenatal care during pregnancy

In normal pregnancy visits to clinics are usually made at the following intervals:

1. Booking — 28 weeks: 4 weekly (probably unnecessarily frequent).
2. 28–36 weeks: 2 weekly.
3. From 36 weeks: weekly.

At each visit the following are recorded:

1. Weight.
2. Result of urine testing for protein and glucose.
3. Blood pressure.
4. Presence or absence of oedema.
5. Fundal height, fetal lie, presentation, attitude, position and engagement or non-engagement of the presenting part in the pelvis.
6. Presence of fetal heart.
7. Also noted should be the amount of liquor, the size of the baby and any sign of abnormality.

The patient is asked if she has any problems and if she has, these are dealt with as far as possible. A vaginal examination is usually carried out at or after 36 weeks to assess the presenting part, the relative size of fetal head and maternal pelvis, and the state of the cervix. About half way through pregnancy those who wish to breast feed (and this should be encouraged) have their breasts examined and are advised about breast care; the most important aspect is teaching the mother to encourage the nipples to become erect and to roll them gently each day between finger and thumb. Those with inverted, small or flat nipples which do not respond may benefit from the use of breast shields. Towards the end of pregnancy it is important to make sure that the patient knows how to recognize when she is in labour and what to do about getting to hospital.

Additional blood tests are usually taken as follows: haemoglobin and rhesus antibodies (if rhesus negative); 28, 34 or 36 weeks. Other investigations such as urinary oestriols, serum placental lactogen (hPL) cardiotocography and ultrasonography are performed routinely in some clinics but not in others. Similarly some women are given fetal movement (kick) charts in the last trimester.

Women who fail to attend the clinic must be contacted and encouraged to keep their next appointment. In case of difficulty it may be helpful to ask the midwife or health visitor to call.

Dental care
This is free in the UK during pregnancy, and women should be encouraged to take advantage of this facility, particularly as gingivitis is common at this time.

Genetic counselling and prenatal diagnosis of fetal abnormality

When there is a history suggesting an increased risk of fetal abnormality genetic counselling should be sought or advised before pregnancy. If this has not been done and a couple are requesting termination or special investigations it should be arranged urgently. With the investigations available the risk of the procedure has to be balanced against the risk and consequences of fetal abnormality, and couples have to consider what they will do if an abnormality is found. The availability of such tests raises major ethical issues and can present prospective parents with very difficult decisions.

Methods of screening (Table 1.1)
Ultrasound (Fig. 1.1) can be used for major abnormalities, which may be identified incidentally when the biparietal diameter is measured. If a skilled operator takes additional time to scan the vertebral column he can also detect neural tube defects. There is no evidence that ultrasound used for obstetric diagnosis is in any way harmful to mother or fetus.

Serum α-fetoprotein
This test is done after 16 weeks and a raised level suggests an open neural tube defect. It is not, however, very reliable because the maturity must be known precisely and up to 19 out of every 20 women with abnormal values subsequently prove to have normal fetuses. For this reason the test needs to be

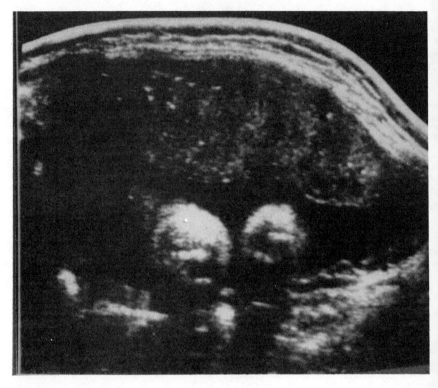

Fig. 1.1 Ultrasound of an anterior wall placenta.

confirmed by a liqour α-fetoprotein estimation and/or ultrasound. The test inevitably induces a severe degree of anxiety in many of those initially found to have an abnormal result.

Liquor α-fetoprotein
A sample of fluid is obtained by amniocentesis with ultrasonic control, to exclude twins and avoid the danger of needling the placenta or fetus, after the 16th week. The result should be available within a day or two. This test is indicated when the serum level is abnormal or if there is a family history of neural tube defect (the risk of recurrence is about 3 per cent when there is already an affected child). The risk under ultrasound control is small and generally accepted to be about 1 per cent for subsequent miscarriage. False positives may occur, for example with exomphalos.

Fetal karyotyping from liquor
Amniocentesis is performed as above and the cells are cultured, though there is a 5 per cent chance that they will not grow. If they do, the result is usually available in approximately three weeks, so that the pregnancy is

Table 1.1 Prenatal diagnosis.

Time	Method	Abnormalities/assessment
Pre-pregnancy	Genetic counselling; diagnosis parental investigations	Risk assessment Counselling
1st Trimester	Ultrasound	Identification of blighted ovum, missed abortion
	Trophoblast biopsy (still experimental)	Chromosome abnormalities, identification of gene dysfunction
2nd Trimester	Amniocentesis: fetal cell culture	Chromosomal abnormalities
	α-fetoprotein and acetyl cholinesterase estimation	CNS defects
	biochemistry of liquor	Metabolic disorders
	cell biochemistry	Immunological disorders
	Maternal blood: serum α-fetoprotein	Screening for CNS defects
	Fetoscopy: visualization of fetal parts	Facial, limb abnormalities
	fetal blood sampling	Haemoglobinopathies, haemophilia
	fetal skin biopsy	Inherited skin disease
	fetal liver biopsy	Liver enzyme abnormalities
	Ultrasound	CNS defects, skeletal/limb defects, tumours, anomalies of the cardiac, gastro-intestinal and urinary tracts, fetal death
	X-ray (rarely used)	Skeletal abnormalities, fetal death

approximately 20 weeks. This is an expensive test, not universally available, and it is therefore offered to those at high risk; usually women above the age of 35 or 37 in whom the risk of Down's syndrome is 1:200 or greater.

This test can also be used when the mother has previously had a baby with a chromosomal disorder or when there is a high risk of a sex-linked disorder, such as muscular dystrophy (Duchenne type). Other unexpected disorders may be detected; counselling and decision are usually not difficult if the abnormality is severe (for example with Edward's or Patau's syndromes), but may be so if the diagnosis is Klinefelter's syndrome (XXY), Turner's (XO) or a mosaic. The liquor and cells may also be used for enzyme detections, tissue typing or examination with a DNA Probe.

Fetoscopy
The fetus can be inspected with an endoscope inserted through the uterine wall and fetal blood samples can be obtained. There is a high risk of abortion, over 5 per cent, and this method of screening is still in its early stages. It is however, valuable for the detection of disorders such as haemophilia and the thalassaemias. This and fetal cell culture may also be used to detect metabolic diseases associated with enzyme abnormalities (e.g. Tay–Sach's disease).

Trophoblast sampling
This takes place in the first trimester and is a new method of examining the

fetal karyotype and other haematological and biochemical characteristics but it is still being developed.

Clincal detection

Finally, fetal abnormality may be suspected clinically later in pregnancy because of polyhydramnios, oligohydramnios or abnormal palpation. In that event ultrasound and/or an X-ray may be helpful. The anxiety and trauma incurred as a result of these tests are considerable and support is needed as well as great care in explaining the significance of any tests or their results.

Minor disorders of pregnancy

This term is misleading because these complaints may in fact be serious in their effects, though fortunately this is rarely the case. They do, however, cause considerable distress and some, for example, interfere severely with sleep.

Nausea and vomiting

This is a common symptom of pregnancy and usually resolves after the first trimester. It is classically worse in the mornings but affects some women more in the evening. Frequent small feeds and avoiding foods which cause nausea may make the symptoms tolerable. Some women find it helpful to have a dry biscuit or drink before getting out of bed in the morning. A few women suffer more severely and require treatment; antihistamines are usually effective though some have a marked hypnotic effect. Avomine (promethazine theoclate) one tablet (25 mg) once or twice daily and Ancoloxin (meclozine hydrochloride 25 mg and pyridoxine hydorchloride 50 mg) one or two tablets at night and in the morning are suitable preparations.

Severe vomiting (hyperemesis) with dehydration, ketosis and weight loss is rare nowadays but will respond to intravenous fluid and antiemetics in hospital. Excessive vomiting is more common with multiple pregnancy and hydatidiform mole. Vomiting in the second trimester may be associated with either of these or with pyelonephritis, though some women suffer throughout pregnancy without any obvious reason for their doing so.

Heartburn

Particularly common in late pregnancy, in those with large babies, hydramnios or multiple births. Avoiding stooping, sleeping with the head and shoulders raised on several pillows and antacids will normally control or at least improve the symptoms. These patients are particularly likely to regurgitate during general anaesthesia.

Constipation

This may be associated with haemorrhoids. Fruit, wholemeal bread and bran will help and, if an aperient is needed, bulk forming laxatives should be advised.

Retention of urine
This occurs rarely in women with a retroverted uterus which as it grows becomes incarcerated within the pelvis usually at about 14 weeks. Treatment is by admission to hospital, catheterization and nursing in the prone position.

Vaginal discharge
This is increased in pregnancy and erosions are very common. If there is any suggestion of infection or pruritus swabs should be taken as well as a cervical smear and appropriate treatment given if infection is diagnosed. The manufacturers advise against using metronidazole in the first trimester but trichomonas can produce severe vaginitis as well as discharge and irritation. *Neisseria, chlamydia* and *candida* all require treatment and can infect the baby at the time of delivery.

Varicose veins
These tend to get worse during pregnancy. Patients should be advised to rest with their legs up and avoid standing as much as possible. Elastic stockings or tights will reduce the deterioration and the risk of thrombophlebitis, as well as protecting against trauma.

Carpal tunnel syndrome (median nerve compression)
This sometimes occurs late in pregnancy and may disturb sleep. If it does, splints, diuretics or local injection of hydrocortisone are usually effective.

Further reading

Hawkins, D.F. Ed (1983). *Human Teratogenesis and Related Problems*. Churchill Livingstone, Edinburgh.
Royal College of Obstetricians and Gynaecologists Working Party (1982). *Antenatal and Intrapartum Care*. Royal College of Obstetricians and Gynaecologists.
Russell, J.K. (1982). *Early Teenage Pregnancy*. Churchill Livingstone, Edinburgh.
Wynn, M and A. (1981). *The Prevention of Handicap of Early Pregnancy Origin*. Foundation for Education and Research in Childbearing, London.

2

Normal labour

Labour is the physiological process by which the uterus contracts, usually at regular intervals and enables the baby to be delivered*. The uterus contracts throughout the pregnancy though this is more marked in some women than in others, and may be painless and hardly noticeable, uncomfortable or actually painful. It is important to define the onset of labour; a combination of regular, painful, sustained contractions usually at intervals of 10 minutes or less with the cervix dilated at least 2 cm. There may be loss of the mucus plug, with or without a little blood, at the onset of labour. Once normal labour has started the contractions increase in strength and frequency until they last up to a minute and occur every 2–5 minutes. Each contraction shortens the muscle fibres of the uterus and some of this shortening is maintained ('retraction') while the cervix is thinned, effaced and dilated. Usually progress is quicker in the latter part of labour i.e. after the cervix is 5 cm dilated than earlier.

The first stage of labour
This lasts from the onset until the cervix is fully dilated.

In the second stage the woman usually feels the urge to bear down; additionally she may have the urge to defaecate and notice more pressure in the pelvis and backache. The rhythm of her contractions and breathing usually changes noticeably. Sometimes the presenting part is visible in the vagina and the anus is dilated at this stage. Any patient who says she wishes to push should be taken seriously because the second stage can be very rapid particularly in multigravid women, although some have the urge to push before full dilatation and this is potentially dangerous. If there is any doubt the problem can be solved by waiting a few minutes during which the patient should 'breathe the contractions away', instead of pushing voluntarily and it is usually quickly apparent if she has reached the second stage. Alternatively a vaginal examination will determine the stage of the cervix accurately. Pushing too early wastes energy and can produce oedema of the cervix or push the presenting part through the incompletely dilated cervix which can then clamp

*See Findlay *Reproduction and the Fetus*, Chapter 8:

down on the baby. The first stage of labour usually lasts between 4 and 12 hours for a primagravida and 1–8 hours for a multigravida. The membranes may rupture before labour is established, at the onset or at anytime thereafter, occasionally remaining intact until the second stage.

Second stage
This lasts from the time of full dilatation of the cervix until the delivery of the baby. It is marked by 'bearing down' or pushing effects with the uterine contractions which lead to expulsion of the baby. In a primigravid patient it usually lasts about one hour while in the normal multigravida it is shorter and varies from a few minutes to an hour.

Third stage
This lasts from delivery of the baby to delivery of the placenta. The uterus contracts after delivery of the baby and the placenta attached to it does not so that the placenta becomes separated in a number of places. Bleeding at these sites helps to separate the two further and the uterus contracts more as the placenta becomes detached. It will then be pushed down into the lower segment and expelled into the vagina. When the placenta descends the cord will lengthen; if the placenta is in the lower segment the uterus will feel hard and round like a ball. A show (a gush of blood) often occurs at the time of separation or with delivery.*

Anatomy

The uterus has grown enormously during pregnancy and during the last trimester the lower segment is formed. This is the lower thinner part of the uterus which stretches during labour while the rest of the muscle contracts and retracts. The cervix softens during pregnancy when it may also be partly dilated and effaced before labour starts. During labour the cervix is taken up

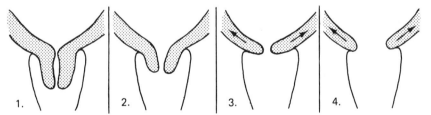

Fig. 2.1 The cervix in pregnancy and labour.

fully, thinned and then dilated (Fig. 2.1). At full dilatation it measures approximately 10 cm across. You will find it helpful to revise the anatomy of the pelvis. The inlet, cavity and outlet are shown in Figure 2.2. The maximum diameters should be noted since the mechanism of labour depends on the widest diameter of the fetal head fitting into the widest diameters of the pelvis.

*For physiological changes at birth see Findlay, *Reproduction and the Fetus*, Chapter 8.

A = True conjugate (average 11.0 cms AP diameter of inlet)
B = Diagonal conjugate (average 12.5 cms)
C = AP diameter of the outlet (average 13.5 cms)

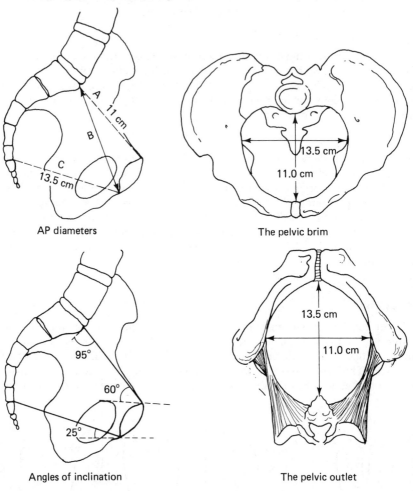

AP diameters

The pelvic brim

Angles of inclination

The pelvic outlet

Fig. 2.2   The pelvis.

Definitions

Lie
The long axis of the fetus described in relation to that of the uterus, usually longitudinal but may be transverse or oblique.

Presentation
The fetal part presenting in or immediately above the cervix. It may be part of the head (vertex, face, brow), shoulder, breech or limb. The vertex is the area between the anterior and posterior fontanelles and the parietal eminences.

Attitude
The head and limbs are usually flexed on the trunk but they can be extended.

Position
The relation of part of the fetus (the denominator) to the pelvis. The denominator is the occiput in a cephalic presentation and the sacrum with a breech presentation. It is normally described as anterior, posterior or lateral.

Station
The level of the presenting part usually described in relation to the ischial spines, though the pelvic brim is an alternative.

The mechanism of labour

It is essential to understand the mechanism by which the fetus passes through the pelvis in order to conduct labour and delivery safely and properly and to understand and recognize what can go wrong. Knowledge of the anatomy indicates what must happen if the fetus is to pass through. A pelvis and fetal 'doll' can be used to work out or demonstrate the series of movements.

Descent   The fetus, and the head in particular, must be pushed down by the contractions and this continues throughout normal labour.

Flexion   Unless the normal sized head is fully flexed or extended it cannot enter the pelvis because it is too big. The normal situation is for the head to flex as it descends with contractions; the suboccipito-bregmatic diameter (9.5 cm) will therefore be the diameter engaging in the brim of the pelvis. (Fig. 2.3).

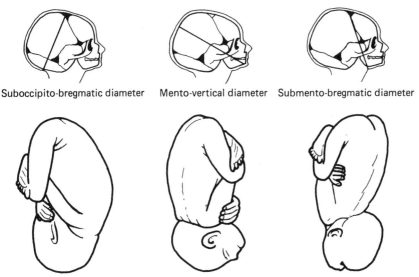

Suboccipito-bregmatic diameter   Mento-vertical diameter   Submento-bregmatic diameter

Flexion (vertex)   Brow presentation   Extension (face)

Fig. 2.3 Diameters of the fetal head and fetal attitude.

Engagement   Engagement means that the widest transverse diameter of the fetal head (the biparietal approximately 9.5 cm) has passed through the pelvic brim and it may occur before or during labour. The widest diameter of the fetal head enters the widest diameter of the pelvic inlet which is the transverse. In some women, notably African multigravidas, the head may not engage until labour is well advanced.

Internal rotation   With a descending flexed head the occiput will reach the pelvic floor first. This floor is like a gutter formed by the *levator ani* muscles which cause the occiput to rotate forwards to lie anteriorly.

Extension and delivery of the head   The head continuing to descend passes below the pubic arch where it can extend as it emerges. The shoulders descend into the brim in the transverse diameter. As they descend further the shoulders rotate like the head to lie in the AP diameter and as they do this the head must rotate also through 90°. This is restitution (the head returning to its normal position in relation to the shoulders) and external rotation (which occurs as the shoulders rotate).

Delivery of the trunk   The anterior and the posterior shoulder deliver and the trunk follows, being flexed laterally to follow the axis of the birth canal.

Variations in the mechanism of labour

Face presentation
The possibility of extension of the head instead of flexion has already been mentioned. In this case the submento-bregmatic diameter (9.5 cm) engages and there is a face presentation which is described according to the position of the chin. Normally the chin rotates anteriorly (mento-anterior) following the same sequence as a vertex presentation and the head is delivered by flexion. If the chin rotates posteriorly delivery is impossible, because the head cannot be delivered by flexion, nor can the head extend any further.

Occipitoposterior position
In some cases the occiput is posterior instead of lateral or anterior and in this position the head does not flex so well and, therefore, may not engage, or may take a long time to do so. If flexion does occur the occiput will reach the pelvic floor first and rotate anteriorly. If the head does not flex well it may still enter the pelvis in the oblique diameter and it can then rotate either anteriorly or posteriorly. In the latter event (persistent occipitoposterior postion) labour is often slow and inefficient and the head is flexed, with the brow and face against the pubis as it is born face to pubis (the face of the baby usually shows the effect of this pressure).

Deep transverse arrest
If the head descends without rotating into the AP diameter it will normally stop because there is insufficient space, usually at the level of the ischial spines. This is an obstructed labour due to failure to rotate.

Incomplete flexion or extension of the head
In these cases the diameter of the fetal skull may be too large for it to enter the pelvis. The extreme example of this is when the mento-vertical diameter (brow) presents; in a normal-sized fetus this is approximately 13.5 cm and engagement is impossible.

Abnormalities of the pelvis

Contraction
This means reduction of one or more of the pelvic diameters, i.e. the whole pelvis, part of it or one diameter may be smaller than normal. The normal female pelvis is described as gynaecoid. The inlet is rounded. Other shapes are:

1. *Android* — triangular flat brim (heart shaped) and convergent side walls with a narrow sub-pubic arch.
2. *Anthropoid* — large brim with long AP diameter, deep cavity with parallel side walls.
3. *Platypelloid* — flat brim with wide transverse diameter and parellel side walls. Rickets in children causes flattening of the pelvis

Congenital abnormalities
1. Naegele pelvis — asymmetric contraction due to absence/poor development of one sacral ala.
2. Roberts pelvis — absence of both sacral alae.
3. High or low assimilation pelvis — the fifth lumbar vertebrae may be fused with the sacrum (giving a deep pelvis) or the first sacral vertebra may be present as an additional lumbar vertebra so that the pelvis is notably shallow.
4. Scoliosis, dislocation of the hip and trauma may also cause asymmetry or contraction of the pelvis.

In assessing the pelvis the important consideration is whether it is adequate for the fetus to be delivered. It is not the size or shape of the pelvis alone that matters, but whether it will allow a specific fetus through, or whether there is disproportion between the head of the fetus (or any other part) and the pelvis.

Examination of the pelvis

The pelvic outlet and cavity can be assessed at vaginal examination, particularly the sacral curve, the prominence of the ischial spines, the subpubic arch and the intertuberous diameter. The inlet cannot be reached but it can be assessed if the presenting part is engaged or will engage (see p. 18). Measurement of the distance from the lower margin of the pubis to the sacral promontory (the diagonal conjugate) gives an indication of the anteroposterior diameter of the brim (this is the obstetric conjugate, usually 11–12 cm and 2 cm less than the diagonal conjugate). The pelvis can be measured radiologically but this is of limited value because: 1. the soft tissues cannot be measured; 2. there is variation in the efficiency of uterine contractions and 3. the size and position of the fetus may vary.

Examination in labour

On admission to hospital in labour the patient should be asked when contractions started, their frequency, strength and length; whether there has been any show and whether her membranes have ruptured. The notes should contain most of the other necessary information required but enquiry about recent events or illness is essential. If for any reason the patient was booked elsewhere or had not booked at all the necessary information, examination and investigations are covered as far as possible.

The temperature, pulse and blood pressure are taken and the abdomen examined. Urine testing for protein and sugar is essential. Detailed preparation for labour varies from hospital to hospital. Shaving or trimming should be minimal and enemas or suppositories are not necessary though many still give them. It is common for the women to have a bath or shower. Vaginal examination is usually performed to determine:

1. The vulva and introitus — size, presence of varices, discharge.
2. Vagina — degree of relaxation, temperature, degree of moisture, presence or absence of blood and or liquor.
3. Fetus — presenting part, position, level in pelvis (station, related to ischial spines), amount of caput (the oedematous part of the head not pressing against the bony pelvis).
4. Cervix — dilatation, thickness, effacement and application to the presenting part.
5. Membranes — intact or ruptured.
6. Liquor — if present, amount and colour.

The pelvis is assessed in relation to the presenting part (which may be pushed down by a contraction or by the examiner's other hand) noting particularly the shape of the sacrum, the promontory if it can be felt, the prominence of the ischial spines, the subpubic angle and the intertuberous diameter.

Observations during labour
These include; maternal temperature, pulse, blood pressure, uterine contractions (frequency, length and strength), urinary output, bowel actions, vomiting, and any other relevant information such as headache, bleeding, rash or visual upset, fetal heart rate or movement.

The progress of labour, assessed by quality and frequency of contraction, descent of the presenting part and dilatation of the cervix (frequency of vaginal or rectal examination varies).

Good nursing care is essential with reassurance, encouragement and explanation as required. The patient should **never** be left alone and the same nurse or midwife should, if possible, attend her throughout labour. Observation and communication will indicate the need for analgesia, intravenous fluids, catheterization or other measures which may be necessary.

The woman may choose to walk about, sit, recline or lie during labour according to how she feels; whether there are any complications and whether she has had any form of analgesia. Lying supine is not advisable because it may compress the inferior vena cava thereby causing hypotension, syncope and reduced uterine perfusion.

In addition to the routine observations the midwife and doctor must watch the general conditions of the patient and her reaction to labour.

After delivery of the anterior shoulder of the baby

An intramuscular injection of an oxytocic is given (usually ergometrine maleate 0.5 mg and oxytocin 5 units). This encourages early contraction of the uterus and separation of the placenta, and reduces the blood loss. Oxytocin alone should be used if the blood pressure is raised. Controlled cord traction is the usual method of delivery of the placenta but it can only be used when the uterus is contracted, otherwise the uterus may be inverted. One hand placed on the uterus supports it and prevents it descending while the other is used to pull the cord down and backwards.

Procedure after the third stage

The following observations should be made and recorded:

1. Condition of the mother including pulse, blood pressure, temperature.

2. Palpation of the uterine fundus for size and contraction. The bladder should be checked and if it is full it should be emptied, normally by the patient's voluntary effort but by catheter if necessary. Urine should be tested for protein.

3. The perineum is inspected for injuries (tears, abrasions and haematomas) and bleeding.

4. The details of the labour and time of birth are recorded. (For examination and resuscitation of the baby see Chapters 3 and 4 respectively).

5. The placenta and membranes are inspected systematically to identify abnormalities such as succenturiate lobe, velamentous insertion of the cord, tumours, infarction, retroplacental thrombosis, calcification and any evidence of tissue retaind in the uterus.

6. The umbilical cord is checked for the presence of knots or other abnormalities, particularly absence of an umbilical artery (which may be associated with a congenital abnormality of the baby).

The episiotomy and any injuries are sutured. The patient is then washed, and settled comfortably in bed with clean clothing and linen as appropriate. Cups of tea are usually welcomed by husband and wife. The general condition of the patient, contraction of the uterus and the amount of vaginal bleeding should be assessed every 15 minutes until the patient leaves the labour ward which she normally does approximately one hour after delivery.

Special care will be required for any patient who has had complications, such as haemorrhage or hypertension, and for any with medical disorders, or who have received special drugs or general anaesthesia. In general patients should not leave the labour ward until their condition is satisfactory and acute problems have been sorted out.

As soon as possible after delivery the mother should hold her baby, let him/her suck at the breast if she wishes, and be given as much privacy with the father as is possible. The clinical care is vital but it must be blended with consideration for the patient and for her need to enjoy the new baby while sharing the occasion with the father.

When the husband or partner is absent or the woman is a single parent she may choose a relative or friend to stay with her in labour.

Repair of episiotomy or vaginal laceration

This is normally carried out with the patient in the lithotomy position, using local infiltration anaesthesia (e.g. lignocaine 1 per cent) if there is not already anaesthesia or if this is inadequate. The vaginal edges are best sutured with a continuous absorbable suture and the deeper perineal tissues with interrupted absorbable sutures. The skin may be repaired with interrupted skin sutures, absorbable or non-absorbable, or by a subcuticular suture. It is important to obliterate the dead space of the perineum and to obtain haemostasis. If any pack or swab is placed in the vagina it must be recorded to ensure that the operator removes it. The repair must not constrict or distort the introitus which should admit 2 fingers comfortably and care should be taken to avoid thin skin edges which may be a cause of dyspareunia later. Episiotomies and repairs are probably the most common sources of complaint among recently delivered women and care should be taken to avoid unneccessary injury and to ensure good healing and minimal discomfort.

The relief of pain in labour

Complaints, often justified, about the pain and stress of labour are still heard, but it is salutary to consider what women must have suffered in the days where operative intervention was impossible or highly dangerous and when there was no effective means of reducing pain. Adequate preparation for childbirth includes preparing a woman for what she is likely to experience in labour and teaching her how to relax, control the pain and cooperate with midwife or doctor in delivering her baby. There are many ways of doing this but none is ideal for everyone, nor does any guarantee a normal delivery. Much emphasis is put on 'natural childbirth' by some women, but they really mean normal delivery with minimal professional involvement. It is important that women's hopes are not raised too high, because unfulfilled expectations may lead the woman to refuse obstetric help to her own or the baby's detriment or to feel guilty about 'her failure'.

It is perfectly possible for a woman to come through a normal labour without the assistance of analgesics; education and relaxation contribute greatly to this, as do the atmosphere in the place of delivery and the confidence of the mother-to-be in her professional assistants.

Pethidine

This is the most widely used parenteral analgesic, given by intramuscular injection in a dose of 50–200 mg. It can cause vomiting and may be prescribed with another drug with sedative and, particularly, antiemetic properties. Any drug which depresses the central nervous system will cross the placenta and similarly affect the baby, in particular depressing respiration and suckling behaviour. For this reason there has been a movement to reduce the dose of pethidine to 50–100 mg and to avoid long acting drugs such as promethazine and diazepam. If possible pethidine should not be given late in the first, or in the second, stage. Some women dislike the sedative action and the feeling it gives them of not being fully in control. Morphine and omnopon have also been used but cause even greater depression of the infant. All these drugs and pethidine can be reversed with naloxone given either to the mother before delivery, or to the baby.

Inhalation anaesthesia

A mixture of 50 per cent oxygen and 50 per cent nitrous oxide (Entonox) is often used when it is too late to give pethidine. It is inhaled as soon as the approaching contraction is recognized so that it is effective at the peak when the patient may need to push. Other gases used include trichlorethylene and methoxyflurane, but these are used less than they were. Nitrous oxide is used because it acts quickly, is safe with oxygen, does not depress respiration in the neonate, and can be controlled by the mother.

Local anaesthesia

1. Local infiltration of the perineum is used before episiotomy.
2. Pudendal block. The pudendal nerve is blocked by injecting local anaesthesia just beyond and below the ischial spine round which the pudendal nerve turns. 10 ml of 1 per cent lignocaine is delivered with a 10 cm needle passed transvaginally or percutaneously (the needle being introduced at a point half way between the anus and the ischial tuberosity, already anaesthetised with a small quantity of lignocaine).

This can be used for forceps deliveries and should be combined with infiltration of the perineum and vulva (ilio-inguinal, genitofemoral nerves and perineal branch of the posterior cutaneous nerve of the thigh).

Epidural nerve block

Local anaesthetic, (lignocaine 1.5 per cent or bupivicaine 0.5 per cent) is injected into the epidural space in the lumbar region. This may be done directly or via a fine catheter which enables the block to be 'topped up' when the effect wears off. This gives excellent pain relief and is particularly valuable in the following situations:

1. Cardiac disease; removes pain, stress and the desire to push in the second stage.
2. Hypertension; reduces or removes painful stimuli and lowers the blood pressure.
3. Premature labour; minimal depressive effect on the fetus.
4. Where control of the delivery is essential or intervention may be required, e.g. twin pregnancy, breech presentation or where elective forceps delivery is indicated.
5. Long labour.

There is danger of acute hypotension; the blood pressure and pulse must be recorded and the patient observed, paticularly for the first 15 minutes. The dura may be punctured and if this is not treated by injection of fluid the patient may suffer a severe headache for several days. Patients with epidural blocks may still vomit. Bladder sensation is lost and the patient may have no

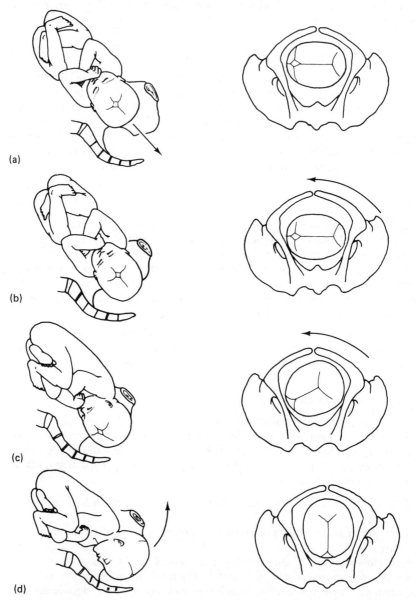

(a)

(b)

(c)

(d)

Fig. 2.4   Passage of the fetal head through the pelvis viewed through the outlet. Note the rotation of the head.

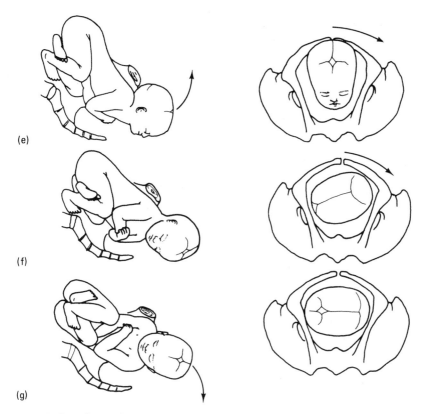

(e)

(f)

(g)

Fig. 2.4 (cont.)

bearing down sensation and require forceps delivery (up to 75 per cent). Some patients are very enthusiastic about epidurals, others dislike the loss of sensation, control or involvement in labour. Occasionally the anaesthetic may not work.

Contraindications include drug sensitivity, local skin sepsis, anticoagulant therapy and antepartum haemorrhage. Caution should be observed in those with a history of back injuries or operations and in those with uterine scars.

Other forms of nerve block include epidural anaesthesia by the caudal route and paracervical block.

General anaesthesia

This is particularly dangerous for the pregnant woman because of the danger of aspiration of regurgitated stomach contents which block the air passages and produce chemical irritation (Mendelson's syndrome). Additionally the drugs given to depress the maternal nervous system will reach and depress the fetus. For this reason general anaesthesia should be avoided if possible and particularly in high risk patients (the obese, those with hiatus hernia and those with full stomachs). The dangers may be reduced by not giving food to patients during labour, administering magnesium trisilicate mixture 15 ml every 4 hours, as well as before any anaesthetic, and cricoid pressure during induction. Such anaesthetics should only be given by experienced anaesthetists with adequate skilled assistance and full equipment to cope with emergencies (e.g. tipping table, suction, and the appropriate endoscopes).

Fetal monitoring

Careful observation of the wellbeing of the fetus used to be restricted to assessment of fetal size, liquor and auscultation of the fetal heart. Now the fetal heart rate, the changes in rate and the variability can be obtained by the use of fetal scalp electrodes or sensors on the external abdomen; simultaneous recordings of the uterine contractions enable us to relate the two and identify lack of variation in the rate, abnormal rates, Type I dips (slowing synchronous with contractions and due to interferences with the feto-placental circulation) and Type II dips (Fig. 12.2, p. 131)(slowing after contractions, and associated with fetal hypoxia). The acid base status can be measured in blood obtained from the fetal scalp during labour, the normal pH being 7.35; when there is hypoxia the pH is below 7.20 indicating that the fetus is in danger. Maternal acidosis may involve the fetus and can be corrected by adminstration of sodium bicarbonate.

The use and value of monitoring are controversial. At present it is generally felt that continuous monitoring should be used selectively in cases when the risk is thought to be above average. Not everyone accepts its value and some women find the equipment disturbing and restrictive. Telemetry permits women to move about while being monitored. It is difficult to believe most would not find it acceptable if they were convinced that it would increase the safety of their baby during labour and delivery. The onus is on the obstetrican and midwife to prove the value, minimize adverse effects, and ensure that patients can make properly informed decisions about monitoring and other potentially controversial matters.

Active management of labour

In days gone by some women used to labour longer than we would consider acceptable; for example 48 hours, whereas now most would regard 12 hours as long enough for any primigravida and too long for some. The causes and consequences of long labour are discussed later. The concept of the active management of labour was introduced as a means of detecting and correcting slow progress. The principles include a careful record of the rate of progress of labour on a chart which may include a line or lines indicating when there is significant delay (Fig. 2.5). The practice includes early rupture of the membranes and stimulation of contractions with intravenous oxytocin when progress is not sustained. Many obstetricians and midwives are firmly convinced that this management benefits mother and child greatly, but others are unhappy at the concept of interference by rupture of the membranes and use of oxytocin. Attitudes and regimes differ but we do not, and should not, see women in prolonged labour in well run obstetrics units nowadays, nor do we see the disasters and long-term complications which resulted from long labour. It is vital that patients understand why we advocate active management in some situations and what is involved since we cannot do anything without their consent. Additionally, intravenous oxytocin should only be given when it is indicated (e.g. when progress is slow) and with appropriate supervision and observation. The use of oxytocin can be dangerous, particularly in women who have had children before (multigravida). In obstructed labour (see p. 134) or in those with very strong contractions due to over stimulation the uterus may rupture.

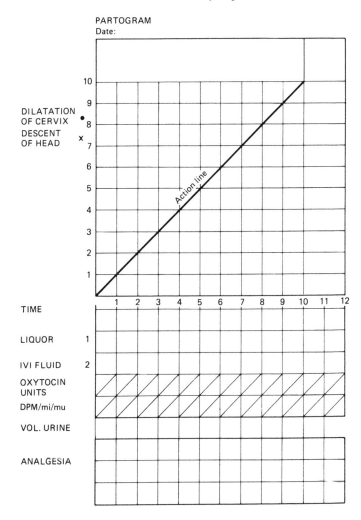

Fig. 2.5

Further reading

Pregnancy Book (1984). Health Education Council, London.
Selwyn Crawford, J. (1982). *Obstetrics, Analgaesia and Anaesthesia: Current reviews in obstetrics and gynaecology No. 1.* Churchill Livingstone, Edinburgh.

3

The normal newborn

N.R.C. Roberton

Mother-child interaction

There is now a large body of evidence to show that in humans, as in mammals and other primates, separating the newborn infant from its mother can have serious adverse effects. The process whereby a mother and her baby get to know each other has been called 'bonding' or better 'attachment'. Failure of attachment can impair relationships between the mother and her baby for many months. Such mothers seem to be less affectionate to their babies and less able to cope with minor problems; breast feeding is less likely to be successful, and the infant is more likely to suffer from failure to thrive or nonaccidental injury in infancy.

In the first hour or two after delivery, healthy infants who are not depressed by drugs or perinatal asphyxia are at their most alert and appealing. Every effort should be made, therefore, to allow the mother and her baby to enjoy each other, and for the first breast-feed to be given at this time. To encourage this, the infant should be left with the parents after delivery, and not snatched away for arcane nursing rituals such as weighing and measuring, and particularly bathing which is not only unnecessary, but is a very effective way of causing neonatal hypothermia.

Thereafter the mother should be allowed to keep the baby in a cot beside her bed, the practice of 'rooming-in', and should be encouraged to care for and feed her own infant whenever needed.

Even without the evidence from research that there are serious sequelae from neonatal mother–child separation, those responsible for medical care in the neonatal period should remember that the mother has waited 9 months to enjoy her newborn baby. To deny her this is cruel, and unless there is some overpowering medical reason for separating them, it should not be done.

Finally, postnatal visiting time should be liberal, other members of the family including siblings, should be able to come in and see and cuddle the new baby.

Infant feeding*

There are several reasons for encouraging the mother to breast-feed her baby.

*See Findlay, *Reproduction and the Fetus*, Chapter 9.

Table 3.1 The advantages of breast feeding

Anti-infection:
    breast milk contains immunoglobulins, complement, lactoferrin, lysosome and white cells; stools stay acid in breast-fed infants inhibiting pathogenic bacteria; lactobacilli become the dominant organisms

Nutritional
Chemical
Emotional/psychological
Food intolerance/allergy — less in breast fed
Cot death — less in breast fed
Convenience/cost — better in breast fed

(Table 3.1). The most important of these from a biological point of view is the prevention of infection, and perhaps preventing allergy and cot death. Although the evidence suggesting that breast-feeding prevents subsequent atopic disease and cot death is controversial. It is important to remember that a major reason for recommending breast-feeding is that it can be an intensely satisfying personal experience for the mother. Breast-feeding is a rare phenomenon; something that is not only cheap and enjoyable, but is actually good for you.

In the 1980s, the infant milk manufacturers have been very successful in changing what is produced by the cow into a milk which has a chemical and nutritional composition that is safe and acceptable for the newborn human. There is no convincing evidence that full term infants come to biochemical or nutritional harm if they are fed on the formulae listed in Table 3.2.

Table 3.2 Chemical and nutritional composition of milk and formulae.

	Cow	Breast	SMA gold cap	Cow and Gate premium	Osterfeed	Aptamil
Carbohydrate (g/100 ml)	4.7	7.4	7.2	6.9	7.0	7.2
Fat (g/100 ml)	3.8	4.2	3.6	3.45	3.81	3.6
Protein (g/100 ml)	3.3	1.1	1.5	1.8	1.45	1.5
(Casein: lactalbumin ratio)	4:1	2:3	2:3	2:3	2:3	2:3
Cals/100 ml	65	70	66	65	68	65
Na mmol/litre	25	6.4	6.4	10	8.3	18
K mmol/litre	36	15	14	15	15	14
Ca mmol/litre	32.5	9	11	12	9	14
PO_4 mmol/litre	32	4.8	10.7	10.0	10.0	11.3
Fe mg/dl	0.15	0.008	1.27	0.65	0.96	0.7
Vit A μg/100 ml	17–38	60	80	80	100	61
Vit D μ/100 ml	0.5	0.8*	1.1	1.1	1.0	1.0
Vit E μ/100 ml	60	350	950	1000	480	600
Folic acid μg/100 ml	3.7	5.2	3.2	3.5	3.4	10

*Water soluble vitamin D

There are disadvantages to breast-feeding (Table 3.3), the most important of which is the transfer of drugs to the infant in pharmacologically active quantities (Table 3.4). A problem which often presents is a mother who is

Table 3.3 Disadvantages of breast feeding.

Few calories for 1st 48 hours:
    important in small-for-dates infants at risk from hypoglycaemia

Maternal discomfort:
    breast engorgement
    cracked nipples
    power of neonatal jaws

Drug passage

Inadequate supply:
    infant fails to gain weight

More frequent feeding:
    may be needed 2–3 hourly
    need night time feeds for longer

Note. Breast feeding alone is not an adequate contraceptive.

Table 3.4 Drugs which enter breast milk.

Absolute contraindication to breast feeding
Antithyroid drugs including radioiodine
Antimetabolites
Narcotics
Ergot
Tetracyclines
Dindevan

Relative contraindication to breast feeding	
Sulphonamides	Reduce bilirubin binding to albumin in infant increasing the risk of kernicterus
Ampicillin	Candidiasis in infant
Nalidixic acid	Haemolysis
Barbiturates, benzodiazepines and phenothiazines	May be sedative
Lithium	Hypotonia in infant
Salicyates in big doses	Platelet function
Oral hypoglycaemic agents	Severe neonatal hypoglycaemia
Anthraquinone laxatives	Diarrhoea in baby
High oestrogen contraceptive pill	Milk production in mother reduced
Diuretics	Diuresis in the infant
Isoniazid	Liver damage

taking one of many drugs acting on the central nervous system such as anticonvulsants, psychotropics and tranquilizers. Apart from Lithium these drugs are however not a routine contraindication to breast-feeding. However, if an infant of a mother taking such drugs becomes sleepy and sedated while breast-feeding, and the drugs cannot be discontinued, then he will have to be bottle fed.

Establishing lactation

There are certain key factors involved in establishing satisfactory lactation*, (Table 3.5), even if the mother is motivated towards breast-feeding her infant,

*See Findlay, *Reproduction and the Fetus*, Chapter 9.

Table 3.5 Factors promoting adequate lactation.

Positive maternal and paternal attitude and adequate prepregnancy education
Antenatal preparation of nipples
Early suckling in labour ward
Avoiding mother infant separation subsequently — for admission to premature baby unit or prohibition of maternal feeding over night in postnatal ward
Demand feeding with rooming-in on the postnatal ward
Frequent suckling 2-hourly acceptable, and promotes prolactin release
Adequate maternal nutrition and hydration
Avoid test weighing — this is a major 'turn off' in mothers
Avoid drugs which might inhibit lactation — oestrogen (the pill)
Avoid maternal stress in the neonatal period

and appropriate antenatal care has been given to ensure that her nipples are not retractile and have been prepared by massage and manipulation for the assault by a set of neonatal jaws.

Two factors which are very important but often forgotten are firstly, the importance of putting the baby to the breast within the first hour after delivery (see above), and secondly the frequency of feeding. Making a mother adhere to a rigid 4-hourly feeding schedule on a postnatal ward is one of the major reasons for lactation failing in a maternity hospital. Breast-fed infants need feeding every 3–3½ hours in the first week or 2, and the postnatal ward routine *must* allow the mothers to feed in this way. Not only does this keep the mother and baby happy, but prolactin production and thus milk formation is stimulated by more frequent suckling. It is also unnecessary to restrict the amount of time an infant spends sucking; contrary to popular belief there is not association between the time spent feeding and problems such as sore or cracked nipples or mastitis.

Bottle feeding babies

Mothers should not be made to feel guilty because they wish to bottle feed. Infants who are bottle fed should be fed on demand, and usually settle quickly into a 4-hourly pattern. The following volumes of milk should be given:

Day 1	60 ml/kg
Day 2	90 ml/kg
Day 3	120 ml/kg
Day 4	150 ml/kg
Day 5	170 ml/kg

Weight gain

All newborn infants lose some weight in the first few days due to fluid loss. Usually they lose about 5 per cent of their birthweight, but it is not abnormal for them to lose up to 10 per cent. After the 4th and 5th day they should start to gain weight; for the first 6 months of life this should average 30 g/day or about 200 g/week.

Keeping babies warm

It is very important to remember that newborn infants can cool off very rapidly if not kept in a warm environment and adequately clothed. Babies whose body temperature falls below 35°C have a considerably higher mortality than those who do not, and this is of greatest importance in the low birthweight infant. Figure 3.1 shows the appropriate temperature at which clothed and naked newborn infants of different birthweights should be nursed.

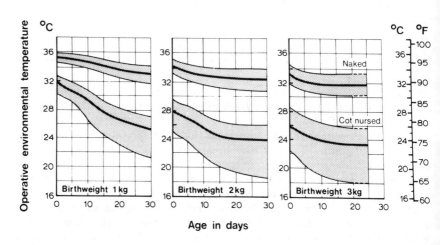

Fig. 3.1 Temperature at which infants weighing 1.0, 2.0 and 3.0 kg should be nursed to maintain a normal body temperature in a draught-free environment at 50% relative humidity. The solid line represents the average temperature, and the hatched area the range of temperatures within which naked or clothed infants can be expected to maintain their body temperature without the expenditure of excess energy. (With permission from Hey, E.N. (1971). The Care of babies in incubators. In *Recent Advances in Paediatrics,* pp. 171–216. Edited by Gairdner, D. and Hull, D. Churchill Livingstone, Edinburgh.)

Prevention of infection

For the reasons given on p. 60 newborn infants are more susceptible to infection than older ones. However they respond to infection with virtually normal cellular and humoral immune responses.

Newborn infants rapidly pick up respiratory tract and gut flora from their environment, primarily from their mothers. She, and indeed other members of the family, are colonized with a largely nonpathogenic, antibiotic-sensitive flora, and other than social cleanliness, and common sense avoidance of overt contagious disease, there is no point in making any attempt to protect full term newborn infants from colonization from these sources.

It is a very different story where hospital staff, nurses, midwives, paediatricians, obstetricians, and even medical students are concerned. We are colonized with unpleasant pathogenic, antibiotic-resistant germs, and we have to come to terms with the fact that we are microbiologically much more unsavoury than the parents, even those fresh from the factory floor or the farmyard. Nevertheless the only important precaution we should take to prevent our flora being transmitted to susceptible neonates in a maternity hospital is rigorous attention to hand washing. Techniques such as gowning and masking are pointless in the routine care of normal neonates.

Umbilical cord care
If infants are going to pick up dangerous organisms from their environment, then the colonization usually starts in the necrotic umbilical stump. An essential part of routine neonatal care is, therefore, preventing umbilical stump sepsis by daily applications of antistaphylococcal or antibiotic sprays, lotions or powders.

Examination of the newborn

All newborn infants should have at least one full physical examination within the first few days of birth. The purpose of this examination is fourfold, to:

1. Identify conditions which require immediate treatment, e.g. buphthalmos or congenital dislocation of the hip.
2. Identify conditions which require long-term supervision and treatment, e.g. cataract or congenital heart disease. These conditions should always be sought neonatally, not only to sustain parents' confidence in their medical attendants, but also because the conditions may be easier to treat if detected at this stage.

Table 3.6 Conditions of no clinical importance which may cause maternal anxiety.

Skin lesions: strawberry naevi
'stork bite'
milia
erythema toxicum
innocent pigmented naevi
epithelial pearls in the mouth
Cephalhaematoma
Subconjunctival haemorrhage
Peripheral and traumatic cyanosis
Tongue tie
Diastasis recti
Protruberant xiphisternum
Hydroceles
Sacral dimple
Umbilical anomalies
Physiological jaundice
Snuffles
Periorbital oedema
Talipes calcaneo-valgus
Vaginal skin tag
Breast enlargement
Hooded foreskin

3. Identify conditions which have important genetic implications, e.g. mongolism or neural tube defects.
4. Note conditions which are in fact variations of normal, but which may be causing the mother anxiety which she is afraid to voice (Table 3.6).

The normal clinical examination should always be carried out in the presence of the mother. It is different from the much more complicated examination designed to evaluate the presence of symptoms in an ill infant. The examination described here is designed to detect important and treatable abnormalities which will not cause symptoms in the neonatal period, and could otherwise pass undetected.

General examination

Obvious external abnormalities such as hare lips, extra digits, birthmarks and club feet will virtually always have been detected by the parents or the nursing staff immediately after delivery. However, a host of minor abnormalities which are of no clinical significance, but may be causing maternal anxieties, may be detected (Table 3.6). The examiner should comment on these to the mother and reassure her about their benign nature.

Cardiovascular system

Is the baby pink? Check the arterial pulses, and in particular the femorals to exclude coarctation of the aorta. Check the heart rate and rhythm. Is the heart on the left, and are the heart sounds normal? Is there a murmur? Remember that most murmurs heard in asymptomatic infants in the first few days of life are of no significance and will disappear.

Respiratory system

So long as the infant is pink and not dyspnoeic and he does not have significant upper or lower respiratory tract disease there is, therefore, no need to do a more detailed examination.

Examination of the abdomen

Many entirely normal infants have up to 2 cm of hepatomegaly and splenomegaly. In the absence of other signs or symptoms these findings are innocent. Always palpate for enlargement of the kidneys and bladder, and note any other masses. Such findings are very rare, but always require immediate investigation.

Examination of the genitalia

Ensure that a full set of external genitalia are present and correct.

Central nervous system

Note the infant's posture, tone and movements. If these are normal, he can suck normally, and he looks at you and follows a moving object, significant neurological abnormalities are highly unlikely to be present. There is nothing to be gained by putting the infant through a series of automatisms such as the Moro response or doing his reflexes.

Always, however, check that the fontanelles are normal in shape, size, number and tension, and measure his head circumference (normal 33–37 cm at term). Examine the infant's eyes to exclude external abnormalities. Ophthalmoscopy is not necessary. Check the vertebral column for scoliosis, midline pits or birthmarks that might suggest intraspinal problems.

Skeletal problems
The single major justification for the routine examination of the neonate is the detection of congenital dislocation of the hip. This is done as shown in Figure 3.2. The infant's flexed leg is held with the femoral trochanters held between the fingers and thumb. In the Ortolani manoeuvre the examiner gently attempts to abduct the hip fully. Failure to achieve this indicates that the hip is dislocated, and a mixture of gentle traction on the leg, plus continued abduction will result in the head of the femur 'clunking' back into the acetabulum. If the Ortalani test is normal, the hip could, however, still be dislocatable. This is tested for by Barlow's manoeuvre, in which the infant's leg is held in the same way as before. While applying gentle traction to try and pull the femur away from the pelvis, an attempt is made by gentle pressure with the thumb over the lesser trochanter to dislocate the femoral head backwards out of the acetabulum.

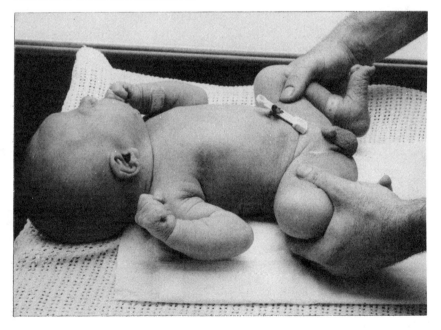

Fig. 3.2 Testing for congenital dislocation of the hip (CDH). The baby's thighs are held as shown. In Ortalani's manoeuvre the legs are fully adducted as shown, thus exlcuding CDH. In Barlow's manoeuvre the legs are held in the position shown and adducted while applying pressure with the thumbs over the lesser tronchanter of the femur. If the hip joint is unstable, the femoral head will dislocate backwards out of the acetabulum as the legs are adducted.

Assessment of the gestational age

This can become a fetish as more and more complex systems are invented. The paediatrician should remember, that in general, his sole purpose in attempting to assess an infant's gestational age postnatally is to establish whether the obstetrician's estimate of the duration of pregnancy is correct, or out by the duration of one menstrual cycle. With this in mind, the following simple examination can be carried out.

Neurological assessment

This is best for infants less than 36 weeks (Table 3.7).

Beyond this period one is dependent on the cutaneous and soft tissue assessment, and the simple assessment system outlined below can be used (Parkin *et al.*, 1976).

Table 3.7 Neurological assesment for infants less than 36 weeks.

Reflex	Stimulus	Positive response	Gestation in weeks if reflex is:	
			Absent	Present
Pupil reaction	Light	Pupil constrictions	<31	29 or more
Glabellar tap	Tap on glabella	Blink	<34	32 or more
Traction response	Pull up by wrists from supine	Flexion of neck or arm	<36	33 or more
Neck righting	Rotation of head of supine infant	Trunk follows head	<37	34 or more

Skin texture

Tested by picking up a fold of abdominal skin between finger and thumb and by inspection:

0 = very thin with gelatinous feel.
1 = thin and smooth.
2 = smooth and of medium thickness, irritation rash and superficial peeling may be present.
3 = slight thickening and stiff feeling with superficial cracking and peeling especially evident in the hands and feet.
4 = thick and parchment-like with superficial or deep cracking.

Skin colour

Estimated by inspection when the baby is quiet:

0 = dark red.
1 = uniformly pink.
2 = pale pink though the colour may vary over different parts of the body, some parts may be very pale.
3 = pale, nowhere really pink except in the ears, lips, palms and soles.

Breast size

Measured by picking up the breast tissue between finger and thumb:

0 = no breast tissue palpable.

1 = breast tissue palpable on one or both sides neither being more than 0.5 cm in diameter.

2 = breast tissue palpable on both sides, one or both being 0.5–1 cm in diameter.

3 = breast tissue palpable on both sides, one or both being more than 1 cm in diameter.

Ear firmness

Tested by palpation and folding of the upper pinna:

0 = pinna feels soft and is easily folded into bizarre positions without springing back into position spontaneously.

1 = pinna feels soft along the edge and is easily folded but returns slowly to the correct position spontaneously.

2 = cartilage can be felt to the edge of the pinna though it is thin in places and the pinna springs back readily after being folded.

3 = pinna firm with definite cartilage extending peripherally and springs back immediately into position after being folded.

The scores obtained on these 4 features are added up and the gestation read off the Table 3.8 below.

Table 3.8 Gestational age (in weeks) estimated from the combined scores of skin texture, skin colour, breast size and ear firmness.

Score	Gestation in weeks
4	34
5	36
6	37
7	38½
8	39½
9	40
10–12	41

Other useful assessments are;

1. Infants with fused eyelids are 26 weeks of gestation or less.
2. In the first hour or two after birth, assess the plantar skin creases; in infants of 36 weeks or less there are one or two transverse plantar creases at the level of the metatarsal heads. By 38 weeks these creases have migrated to the mid point of the sole, and by full term they have reached the heel.

Neonatal biochemical screening

Currently in the UK all newborn infants have a Guthrie Test to exclude phenylketonuria. A drop of capillary blood is collected on the 6th day of life on a piece of absorbent paper, and the phenylalanine level is measured. Infants with abnormally high values are recalled for further testing. In addition, in many parts of the country, a test is done on an identical blood sample to exclude hypothyroidism by measuring blood thyroxine and/or TSH.

Circumcision

Male circumcision is a barbaric ritual for which there is never any medical indication in the neonatal period. It should be viewed with the same abhorrence as female circumcision.

Further reading

Parkin J.M, Hey E.N., and Clowes J.S. (1976). Rapid assessment of gestational age at birth. *Archives of Disease in Childhood* **51**, 259–263.

4

Resuscitation of the neonate

N.R.C. Roberton

Physiology

The sequence of events in neonatal asphyxia has been studied in newborn animals delivered in good condition by caesarean section, and then asphyxiated before the onset of breathing by sealing their heads in a bag of saline. After a few shallow 'breaths' without achieving any gas exchange, the animals stop 'breathing' and enter primary apnoea. After one to two minutes in primary apnoea the animals usually start to gasp with increasing frequency and vigour, though primary apnoea may last for up to 10 minutes. Gasping lasts for 5 to 10 minutes after which the animals make no further spontaneous respiratory efforts (Fig. 4.1).

The heart rate falls rapidly after birth, stays constant or may rise slightly in primary apnoea and early in the phase of gasping, but then slows. Cardiac activity continues for 10 minutes or more after the last gasp. The period between the last gasp and cardiac arrest is known as secondary or terminal apnoea. The changes in blood pressure parallel those in heart rate. By the end of terminal apnoea, the $PaCO_2$ exceeds 13.5 kPa (100 mmHg), the pH is less than or equal to 6.6, and the PaO_2 is unrecordable. Brain damage is only likely in human infants who have reached the stage of terminal apnoea.

If the bag of saline is removed during primary apnoea, after 1–2 minutes the animal will gasp and develop regular respiration. If it is removed when the animal is making respiratory movements or gasping, air will enter the lungs, the blood gases will improve and regular respiration will start. In terminal apnoea, spontaneous respirations are never established when the bag is removed. To resuscitate such an animal positive pressure ventilation must be used and if the heart rate is very slow (or has stopped), external cardiac massage will be necessary.

There is no reason to suppose that the human neonate behaves differently, and his behaviour at delivery will depend on the severity of the preceding intrapartum asphyxia and the degree of drug depression. With a pH greater than 7.25, he will be in the phase of primary apnoea or gasping and regular respirations will soon start. With a lower pH, down to 7–7.10, or with heavy sedation, primary apnoea may be prolonged or the gasping may be insufficient to establish alveolar ventilation; still more severe intrapartum asphyxia will produce an infant in terminal apnoea. In both cases active resuscitation will be required.

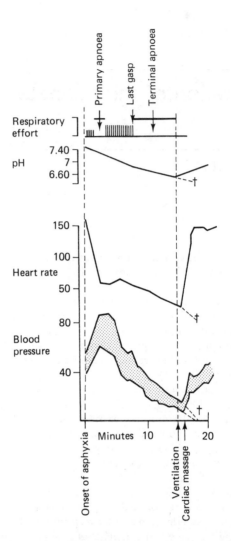

Fig. 4.1   Physiological changes during asphyxia and resuscitation of newborn monkeys. (Adapted from Dawes, G.S. *et al.* (1963). *Journal of Physiology* **169**, 167.)

Assessment of asphyxia

The Apgar score

This score was devised by Dr. Virginia Apgar in 1953 and is based on the evaluation of five clinical features at one minute of age (Table 4.1). However it has limitations, since the physiological significance of the variables scored differs, and the one minute score is a rather poor indicator of the degreee of intrapartum asphyxia. Ideally the infant's condition is assessed as quickly

Table 4.1 Apgar score.

Clinical feature	0	Score 1	2
Heart rate	0	<100	100+
Respiration	Absent	Gasping or irregular	Regular or crying lustily
Muscle tone	Limp	Diminished, or normal with no movements	Normal with active movements
Response to pharyngeal catheter	Nil	Grimace	Cough
Colour of trunk	White	Blue	Pink

after delivery as possible, and the findings recorded in detail in the notes. The response to resuscitation should then be continued as a narrative.

What really matters is whether a newborn baby starts to breathe promptly or not. If the baby does, everything will probably be alright, though occasionally apnoea occurs after a short period of regular respiration. If the baby does not start to breathe, the crucial question is whether or not the apnoea is primary or terminal, since in the former it is reasonable to pursue an expectant policy for 1–2 minutes, inflicting peripheral stimuli in an attempt to initiate respiration. In terminal apnoea, the quicker intermittent positive pressure ventilation (IPPV) is started, the smaller the risk of subsequent brain damage.

About 5 per cent of all newborn infants are in primary apnoea at 1–2 minutes of age. They are in reasonable clinical condition with a heart rate near 100, and have good peripheral perfusion and body tone, although cyanosed and apnoeic (i.e. Apgar 5–6). Approximately 0.5 per cent of all newborn infants are in terminal apnoea and are pale and apnoeic with little or no body tone or reflex response, and have a more profound bradycardia (i.e. Apgar 1–3). However, in many babies who are apnoeic at two minutes of age, it is impossible to be sure whether they are in primary or terminal apnoea, particularly when the mother has been given drugs, and it is safest to treat all such infants as though they are in terminal apnoea.

All neonatal resuscitation should be done on a properly equipped trolley which has on it all the equipment for neonatal resuscitation, and also a large stop clock with a sweep second hand so that during the crisis period accurate timing of events is possible.

Initial assessment of the infant

Start the clock the moment the baby is free from the mother's body (not when the cord is clamped). As soon as the baby is on the resuscitation trolley assess the 5 components of the Apgar score. For heart rate, listen with a stethoscope, do not feel the cord as all you will feel is your own heart beat pounding away in your finger tips.

The baby will fall into one of 4 groups:

1. Fit and healthy, bawling lustily.
2. Not breathing too well, perhaps in primary apnoea but no immediate need for panic (5 per cent).
3. Obvious terminal apnoea; pale, limp and apnoeic, heart rate less than 80 (0.2–0.5 per cent).
4. 'Dead' but resuscitatable (less than or equal to 0.1 per cent, Cardiac arrest).

1. Fit and healthy

Leave this baby alone! Do not suck him out, since this traumatizes the pharynx, and is a powerful vagal stimulus provoking a reflex bradycardia. Vigorous suction is based on the frequently held misconception that what is coming out of the baby's mouth is inhaled liquor. It is not; it is pulmonary fluid which has been in the lungs prior to birth, and will do no harm if it stays there a few moments longer. If the upper airway is full of meconium or blood the infant should be laryngoscoped and his mouth, larynx and trachea aspirated under direct vision.

The infant should be dried and wrapped in a warm blanket to minimize heat loss, given a dose of vitamin K (see page 71) and given to his mother (see page 28).

2. Not breathing too well

There is no immediate panic, follow the diagram in Fig. 4.2. Most of these infants respond to bag and mask resuscitation. Their clinical condition at birth and their prompt response to resuscitation (see below) indicates that they were in primary apnoea.

Note

Bag and mask ventilation is difficult to do effectively, particularly in the infant who has never breathed and cleared his lungs of liquid. To do it effectively, you must have a tight seal where the mask is applied to the infant's face. Slightly extend his neck and hold his jaw and tongue forward: an oropharyngeal airway may help.

When resuscitating a baby by any method, make sure that the chest is moving and the lungs are being inflated. If this is not happening you are doing something wrong, and if you are using bag and mask resuscitation it is probably safest to progress to intubation.

If you have no bag and mask, or it is not working, and intubation is not possible, mouth to mouth (plus nose) resuscitation works very well, but put in an oral airway and remember to extend the infant's neck.

Only give naloxone (1 ml = 0.01 mg) after you have established respiration by whatever means necessary. *NEVER* give it to an apnoeic infant. Naloxone is best given intravenously. In situations where the infant is pink but breathing irregularly, it is perfectly acceptable to give the naloxone intramuscularly while watching the infant carefully until the drug begins to work.

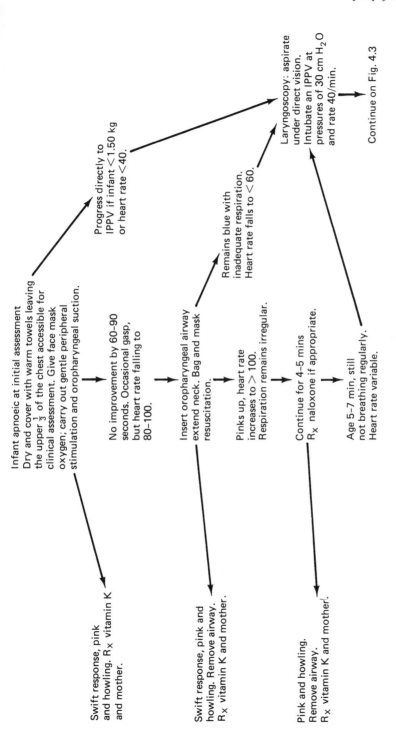

Fig. 4.2 Initial stages in the resuscitation of the apnoeic neonate. (Reproduced from *A Manual of Neonatal Intensive Care* by Roberton, N.R.C. (1981). Edward Arnold, London.)

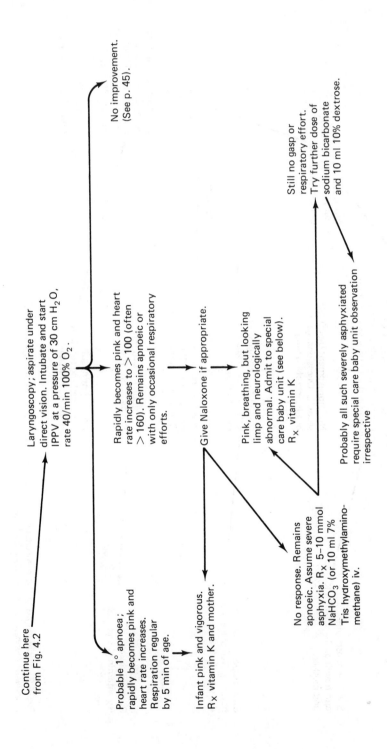

Continue here
from Fig. 4.2

Probable 1° apnoea;
rapidly becomes pink and
heart rate increases.
Respiration regular
by 5 min of age.

Infant pink and vigorous.
R$_X$ vitamin K and mother.

Laryngoscopy; aspirate under
direct vision. Intubate and start
IPPV at a pressure of 30 cm H$_2$O,
rate 40/min 100% O$_2$.

Rapidly becomes pink and heart
rate increases to > 100 (often
> 160). Remains apnoeic or
with only occasional respiratory
efforts.

Give Naloxone if appropriate.

No response. Remains
apnoeic. Assume severe
asphyxia. R$_X$ 5–10 mmol
NaHCO$_3$ (or 10 ml 7%
Tris hydroxymethylamino-
methane) iv.

Pink, breathing, but looking
limp and neurologically
abnormal. Admit to special
care baby unit (see below).
R$_X$ vitamin K

Still no gasp or
respiratory effort.
Try further dose of
sodium bicarbonate
and 10 ml 10% dextrose.

Probably all such severely asphyxiated
require special care baby unit observation
irrespective

No improvement.
(See p. 45).

Fig. 4.3 Later stages of resuscitation of the apnoeic neonate. (Reproduced from *A Manual of Neonatal Intensive Care* by Roberton, N.R.C. (1981). Edward Arnold, London.)

3. Obvious terminal apnoea

About 0.2–0.5 per cent of all deliveries are in this state. Such a baby is severely asphyxiated.

He will never breathe on his own unless you start him off. The longer you delay, the more profound the biochemical and physiological abnormalities, and the greater the likelihood of brain damage. Expeditious action is essential; follow the flow diagrams in Fig. 4.2 and 4.3.

If gasping or respiration does not start after a single dose of bicarbonate, get blood gas and glucose measurements if possible before speculatively administering further drugs.

Always note the time between the onset of resuscitation and the onset of respiration since this gives an indication of the severity of asphyxia; the longer the time, the more severe the asphyxia, and the greater the likelihood of both short term and long term neurological problems.

4. 'Dead'

If the obstetrician is certain that the fetal heart was heard up to 10 minutes pre-delivery, it is always worth attempting to resuscitate the fresh, apparent stillbirth. For one thing, some infants respond very quickly and dramatically to resuscitation and are vigorous and active by 5–10 minutes of age. These were either not stillbirths (i.e. had very quiet and slow heart sounds not detected by the panicking paediatrician), or had undergone a sudden acute asphyxial or vagal stimulus that caused cardiac arrest, without previous prolonged and potentially brain damaging asphyxia. Even for the infant who has undergone such asphyxia, the neurological outcome in survivors is surprisingly good (Scott 1976).

When confronted with a fresh stillbirth give six to eight beats of external cardiac massage (ECM), and then intubate the baby and proceed as in the post intubation section of Fig. 4.3 give 10 mmol bicarbonate and continue the ECM and IPPV.

If there are still no signs of life give a further 10 mmol of sodium bicarbonate plus 10 ml intravenous 10 per cent dextrose, 1–2 ml 10 per cent calcium gluconate, and 0.5 ml of 1/1000 adrenaline in that order. If these fail repeat the sodium bicarbonate and give intracardiac adrenaline. If there is still no response, the infant will be 8–10 mintues old, neurologically intact survival will not be possible, and resuscitation should therefore be abandoned.

Problems with resuscitation

The infant who does not respond to IPPV

A few infants will remain blue, apnoeic, and bradycardiac despite the above routine. In some cases the reason will be obvious e.g. gross hydrops or severe skeletal abnormalities.

In infants who are externally normal in appearance the reason for the poor response to resuscitation is commonly a technical error in resuscitation. Therefore check:

1. Is the endotracheal tube in the correct place, and not in the oesophagus?

2. Are the lungs being adequately inflated? Inadequate inflation is particularly common when using bag and mask ventilation.

3. Is the endotracheal tube too small: a common mistake? A 3.0 or 3.5 mm tube should always be used.

If technical errors can be excluded:

1. Is the asphyxia more severe than the initial clinical assessment suggested? Give a few beats of ECM and 5–10 mmol (5–10 ml of 8.4 per cent solution) of intravenous sodium bicarbonate plus 5–10 ml of 10 per cent dextrose and continue IPPV. If possible transfer the baby to the neonatal unit for arterial catherization.

2. Is the infant developing severe RDS? Increase the inflating pressure to 35 cm H_2O if possible and increase the rate. This virtually always improves the infant enough to allow transfer to the neonatal unit.

3. Is the infant very pale? Consider fetal haemorrhage; infants may lose more than half their blood volume as a feto–maternal bleed, or from an injury to the placenta or a cord vessel. If the history is suggestive, and the pallor seems due to anaemia, give 15–20 ml/kg of fresh uncross-matched O negative blood at once over ten minutes. This will usually improve the baby enough for him to be transferred to the neonatal unit where a more accurate assessment can be made.

4. Is there a diaphragmatic hernia, suggested by mediastinal shift, poor air entry on the left side (the usual side of the hernia) and a scaphoid abdomen? Get a chest X-ray.

5. Is there a pneumothorax? This can occur spontaneously or as a result of over vigorous IPPV, especially if too small an endotracheal tube has been pushed down into a segmental bronchus. If the infant is deteriorating, insert a wide bore needle into the second intercostal space in the mid clavicular line. Always consider pneumothorax, since if the conditions listed above are excluded very little that is treatable is left.

6. Is there some lung malformation such as the pulmonary hypoplasia of Potter's syndrome (renal agenesis, pulmonary hypoplasia, odd facies, low set floppy ears and postural limb deformities p. 72)? The condition is fatal.

The meconium stained infant

Meconium *staining* does not matter. Inhalation of meconium does. A paediatrician should attend all deliveries where there is meconium stained liquor. Even if vigorous at birth, such an infant should be laryngoscoped, meconium stained liquor aspirated from his mouth and pharynx, and the trachea inspected to see if he has inhaled any meconium. If he has, the trachea should be sucked out under direct vision. If large amounts of meconium have been inhaled, bronchial lavage should be considered.

Further reading

Roberton, N.R.C. (1981) *A Manual of Neonatal Intensive Care*. Edward Arnold London.

Scott, H.M. (1976). Outcome of very severe birth asphyxia. *Archives of Disease in Children* **51**, 712–16.

5

The abnormal newborn

N.R.C. Roberton

Definitions

Preterm
A neonate, irrespective of birthweight born before 37 completed weeks of pregnancy, timed from the first day of the last menstrual period.

Low birthweight
The 6.0–7.0 per cent of all low birthweight infants weighing less than 2.50 kg at birth. Many premature neonates as defined above weigh more than this; conversely, about 33 per cent of infants weighing less than 2.50 kg at birth are more than 37 weeks gestation.

Very low birthweight (VLBW)
Although there is no internationally accepted definition of such babies, by

Table 5.1 Illnesses to which preterm infants are particularly susceptible

Respiratory distress syndrome.
Chronic lung disease:
    Recurrent apnoea
    Wilson–Mikity Syndrome
    Bronchopulmonary dysplasia
Patent ductus arteriosus
Jaundice
Metabolic disturbances:
    Hypoglycaemia
    Hypocalcaemia
    Hyponatraemia/hypernatraemia
    Hypothermia
Intraventricular haemorrhage
Anaemia
Infection:
    Pneumonia
    Meningitis
    Septicaemia
    Urinary tract
    Skin
Necrotising enterocolitis

common assent this term applies to the 0.8–1.5 per cent of all neonates weighing less than 1.50 kg at birth. A large proportion of all serious illness, and two-thirds of all neonatal deaths not associated with malformations occur in this group of infants (Table 5.1).

Postmaturity
A neonate, irrespective of birthweight born after the 42nd week of gestation.

Small-for-dates
These are babies whose birthweight falls below some predetermined value at a given gestational age (Fig. 5.1). Some authorities choose the 3rd centile others the 5th or 10th centile, and others minus 2 standard deviations of the normal birthweight for the gestation (Table 5.2). Small-for-dates infants can be either

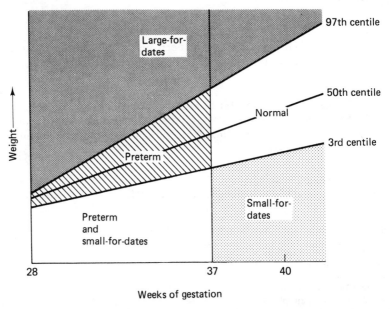

Fig. 5.1 Different groupings of newborn infants. (Reproduced from *A Manual of Neonatal Intensive Care* by Roberton, N.R.C. (1981). Edward Arnold, London.)

Table 5.2 Birthweights (g) for definition of small-for-dates.

Gestation	− 2sd approx 3rd centile (g)	5th centile (g)	10th centile (g)
36	1890	2130	2380
37	2120	2310	2560
38	2335	2470	2710
39	2500	2590	2830
40	2560	2680	2920
41	2615	2740	2980
42	2555	2780	3010

full-term, or postmature (Fig. 5.1). As a group they are at risk from intrapartum asphyxia (p. 39), and once delivered are prone to hypoglycaemia (p. 70). Many malformed infants are small-for-dates.

Respiratory disease in the neonate

Respiratory illness is very common in newborn babies, 2–3 per cent of all infants develop respiratory problems in the first few hours of life. In preterm infants, by far the commonest cause is respiratory distress syndrome.

Respiratory distress syndrome (RDS)

This is caused by lack of surfactant, and is commoner in the more premature the infant (Fig. 5.2). It is also common in infants who have suffered perinatal

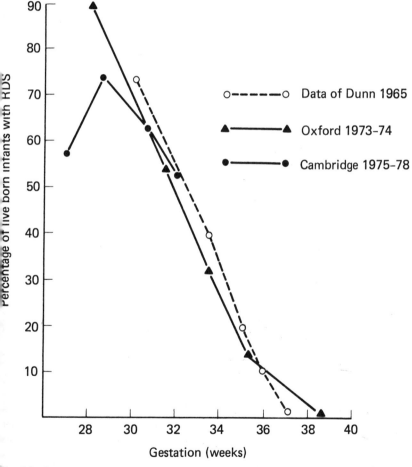

Fig. 5.2 Relation between respiratory distress syndrome (RDS) and prematurity. Reproduced from *A Manual of Neonatal Intensive Care* by Roberton, N.R.C. (1981). Edward Arnold, London.)

asphyxia. In infants over 34 weeks gestation RDS is uncommon unless the mother is a poorly controlled diabetic, or the infant is delivered by caesarean section before the onset of labour.

The lung histology in infants dying from RDS shows widespread atelectasis and the terminal airways are lined with a homogeneous eosinophilic hyaline membrane, hence the alternative name for this condition, hyaline membrane disease.

Symptoms and signs
The 3 cardinal clinical features of RDS which always develop within 4 hours of delivery are:

1. Respiratory rate greater than 60/min.
2. Grunting — expiration against the closed glottis with sudden release of the gas from the lungs, hence the grunt.
3. Intercostal, subcostal and sternal retraction — respiratory distress.

The chest X-ray of such infants shows widespread atelectasis with a reticulo-granular (snowstorm) pattern, and with the air-filled airways standing out against this background giving an air-bronchogram.

Table 5.3 Causes of respiratory disease in first few hours of life.

Surfactant deficient RDS (synonym hyaline membrane disease).
Pneumonia
Aspiration syndrome (meconium aspiration)
Severe asphyxia (hyperventilation due to metabolic acidaemia)
Heart failure (congenital heart disease, myocardial damage)
Pulmonary haemorrhage
Pneumothorax
Congenital malformations in the chest (Table 5.6)
Transient tachypnoea
Persistent fetal circulation
Upper airway obstruction (choanal atresia, Pierre–Robin syndrome)
Neuromuscular disorders (diaphragmatic paralysis, congenital myopathy)

Differential diagnosis
There are many causes of respiratory difficulty coming on in the first few hours of life (Table 5.3). These can usually be differentiated by their clinical features, the history of the delivery, perinatal events and the chest X-ray (Table 5.4). It is however usually impossible to exclude infection as the cause of the infant's respiratory distress, for although analysis of pharyngeal or gastric aspirate for surfactant confirms the diagnosis of surfactant deficient RDS, it fails to exclude coexistent infection.

...ial diagnosis of RDS. From *A Manual of Neonatal Intensive Care* by Roberton, N.R.C. (1981). Edward Arnold, London.

Condition	Gestation	Clinical signs	History	X-ray
Respiratory distress syndrome	Prem > mature	Dyspnoea	Prem delivery. asphyxia. L:S ratio < 2:1	Reticulogranular: air bronchogram
Meconium aspiration	Mature	Distended chest, meconium-stained skin, nails and cord	Meconium-stained liquor. Birth asphyxia. Meconium in trachea at resuscitation.	Streaky atelectasis. Over-expanded lung.
Following intrapartum asphyxia ± other aspiration e.g. liquor, blood	Mature	Usually dyspnoea only: neurological abnormalities	Perinatal asphyxia requiring IPPV	Slightly streaky only
Transient tachypnoea of the newborn	Mature > prem	Tachypnoea, Little grunting	Non-contributory	Fluid in fissures ↑ vascular markings
Massive pulmonary haemorrhage	Mature > prem	Blood welling up trachea or endotracheal tube	Usually severe birth asphyxia. Fluid overload. Hypothermia	opacity, 'white out'
Congenital pneumonia	Any	Sometimes pyrexia and leucocytosis. Hypotonia, early jaundice and apnoea	Infection in mother, prolonged rupture of membranes, smelly liquor.	Usually more blotchy than RDS but may have a bronchogram
Congenital malformation				
a) Diaphragmatic hernia	Mature > prem	Scaphoid abdomen	Nothing abnormal detected	Diagnostic — guts in thorax.
b) Potters syndrome	Usually < term	Potters facies, oligohydramnios, amnion nodosum	Nothing abnormal detected	White out, very small lungs
c) Other malformations	Usually mature	Dyspnoea	Nothing abnormal detected	Diagnostic changes e.g. cysts, emphysema; agenesis
d) Hydrops	Any	Hydrops obvious	Variable	Clinically obvious. Effusions may appear as white out
Pneumothorax	Usually mature if < 4 hours	Hyperresonant, swollen abdomen. Transillumination +ve	May be birth asphyxia → IPPV	Diagnostic
Congenital heart disease	Usually mature if < 4 hours	Other signs heart failure — big liver and heart. Slaty grey cyanosis odd ECG. Murmur.	Nothing abnormal detected	Big heart. Oligaemic or hyperaemic lungs
Persistent fetal circulation	Usually mature	None of heart disease profound cyanosis. ECG normal.	Often mild asphyxia	Chest x-ray often surprisingly normal

Abbreviations: RDS, respiratory distress syndrome; ECG, electrocardiogram; L:S, lecithin: sphingomyelin; and IPPV, intermittent positive pressure ventilation.

Treatment

There is no specific treatment for RDS; the aim of therapy is, therefore, to keep the infant alive until he resynthesizes his own surfactant. This begins 36–48 hours after delivery and if there are no complications the infant usually recovers completely by 5–7 days of age.

Since, in infants with severe RDS, excessive handling by the nursing, medical and paramedical staff may cause rapid deterioration in the infant's condition (Fig. 5.3) it is desirable for all such infants to have the heart rate, respiration, blood pressure and temperature measured electronically to avoid disturbance. All these monitoring devices should be set up as soon as possible after the infant is admitted to the neonatal unit.

All infants should also have an indwelling umbilical arterial catheter for fluid administration and frequent blood sampling particularly for blood gas analysis. Ideally an umbilical artery catheter should be used which has a PaO_2 electrode built into its tip to give a continuous PaO_2 record. Although occasional samples for analysis can be obtained by peripheral arterial

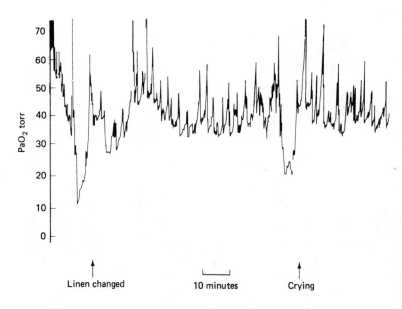

Infant N. M.51227 B.Wt 3.8 kg IRDS on CPAP

Fig. 5.3 Adverse effects of handling an infant with respiratory distress syndrome. (Reproduced from *A Manual of Neonatal Intensive Care* by Roberton, N.R.C. (1981). Edward Arnold, London.)

puncture, this should only be used for initial assessment if the severity of the illness is in doubt, or in mild cases of RDS whose condition is not affected by excessive manipulation.

The basic components of care are:

1. Efficient monitoring (see above).
2. Keep the baby warm; (p. 32) apart from the obvious disadvantages of hypothermia, surfactant function is impaired at low body temperatures.
3. Maintain hydration and normal electrolyte homeostatsis. Some infants with severe RDS have a paralytic ileus, and most need intravenous fluids. Initially, 5–10 per cent glucose with appropriate electrolyte supplements is usually used, and is infused at 60–100 ml/kg/24 h.
4. Keep the blood volume and blood pressure normal (BP greater than 35–40 mmHg systolic, PCV greater than 40 per cent) by infusions of plasma, albumin, whole blood, or occasionally Dopamine.
5. Keep the pH greater than 7.25. If 2, 3 and 4 above are done properly, metabolic acidaemia rarely develops; if it does, infusion of bicarbonate should be given at 0.5 mmol/min.
6. Prevent infection, particularly with the group B streptococcus (p. 32). This cannot usually be excluded in the first 24–48 hours of life in infants with respiratory distress, so give penicillin to all such infants; if IPPV is needed add an aminoglycoside.
7. Nutrition; by 2–3 days of age most infants will tolerate naso-gastric tube milk feeds. If they do not, consider intravenous nutrition.
8. Keep the PaO_2 normal, between 8–12 kPa (60–90 mmHg). This is done at first by increasing the oxygen concentration to 60–70 per cent, but if the infant remains hypoxic in this concentration of oxygen, continuous positive airways pressure (CPAP) using a single or double nasal prong should be used. If this does not prevent hypoxia IPPV is required.

A problem unique to the preterm neonate is retrolental fibroplasia caused by blood with too high a PaO_2 perfusing the retina, too high probably being greater than 16–20 kPa (120–150 mmHg). The high PaO_2 causes capillary spasm, retinal ischaemia and then vascular proliferation progressing to retinal distortion, detachment and subsequent blindness. It is virtually limited to infants less than 32 weeks gestation and 1.50 kg birthweight. Hyperoxaemia is therefore as damaging to the preterm infant as hypoxaemia, and is one of the main reasons why the PaO_2 must be meticulously controlled between 8–12 kPa.

Results
Infants weighing more than 1.50 kg or of more than 30 weeks gestation rarely die from RDS and its complications. In smaller infants, the mortality remains 20 per cent even in a specialized unit.

Sequelae
Most infants make a complete recovery; in a small number their lungs are damaged by the IPPV causing a condition known as bronchopulmonary dysplasia. These infants may remain breathless with abnormal lung function

for 1–2 years but thereafter they are usually alright. In addition, all infants who develop RDS, particularly those with bronchopulmonary dysplasia have an increased incidence of serious lower respiratory tract illness in the first year of life.

Neurological handicap is rare in survivors who weigh more than 1.50 kg at birth but occurs in 10–15 per cent of survivors whose birthweight is less than this.

Other serious respiratory disease in the neonate

Meconium aspiration

This usually occurs in infants of more than 36 weeks gestation since preterm infants rarely pass meconium in utero. The condition is largely preventable by thorough aspiration of all meconium present in an infant's pharynx, larynx and trachea immediately after delivery.

Once meconium gets into the lungs it causes three problems: 1. airway blockage and air trapping by a 'ball-valve' effect; 2. an irritant chemical pneumonitis and 3. a predisposition to lung infection.

Infants with meconium aspiration present within an hour or two of birth and the diagnosis is rarely in doubt. They should be treated like infants with RDS, but always must be given antibiotics, and severe cases usually need IPPV.

Transient tachypnoea of the newborn

This term describes a group of term infants who remain very breathless (respiratory rates 100–120/min) for 24–48 hours after being delivered, often after a transient period of grunting and retraction at much slower respiratory rates. The chest X-ray shows an increase in lung vascular markings, and the condition is attributed to delayed clearance of the fetal lung liquid. The treatment is the same as that for infants with mild RDS. No infant should die of transient tachypnoea of the newborn, and it is rare for one to need more than 40 per cent oxygen to keep his PaO_2 normal.

Airleaks, pneumothorax, pneuomediastinum, pulmonary interstitial emphysema

Following alveolar rupture in neonates air tracks along the bronchovascular bundles to the mediastinum forming a pneumomediastinum. In infants with severe RDS on IPPV, multiple small leaks may occur in this way, but the gas is trapped in the lung parenchyma causing the condition known as pulmonary interstitial emphysema (PIE)(Fig. 5.4).

Although the leaked air may stay within the lung parenchyma or in the mediastinum it commonly ruptures into the pleura causing a pneumothorax. Occasionally pneumothorax and pneumomediastinum may be diagnosed in the first hour or two of life in infants who have no other lung disease; this is most commonly seen in infants who required active resuscitation by IPPV after delivery. However most pneumothoraces occur in infants with lung disease; they develop spontaneously in 5–10 per cent of infants with RDS and meconium aspiration, and the incidence rises to 40 per cent in such infants who require long-term IPPV.

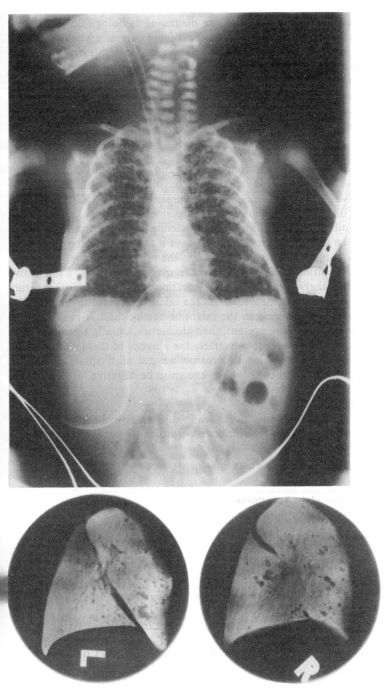

Fig. 5.4 (a) X-ray of a neonate with respiratory distress syndrome (RDS) showing pulmonary interstitial emphysema (PIE), and (b) postmortem demonstration of PIE.

All these conditions with air leaks are diagnosed radiologically, and must always be excluded in any infant in the first few hours of life who develops clinical signs of respiratory difficulty or in any neonate with established lung diseases such as RDS or meconium aspiration, whose condition deteriorates. There is no treatment for PIE and pneumomediastinum other than giving oxygen and keeping the infant alive until the air reabsorbs. Virtually all pneumothoraces require drainage, with connection of the chest tube to an underwater-seal drain.

Pneumonia
Unlike most of the other conditions in Table 5.4 pneumonia can present at any time in the neonatal period, and is the likely diagnosis in an infant over 6 hours of age who develops a respiratory illness. Therefore, all infants who develop lung disease after 6 hours of age must have cultures taken and be started on antibiotics, penicillin or flucloxacillin plus an aminoglycoside, which should be continued for at least 10 days if the cultures are positive.

Pneumonia may also occur in infants less than 6 hours of age, and is the likely cause of respiratory illness at this age in the presence of: 1. a suggestive history in the mother (pyrexia, vaginal infection etc.,); 2. a positive Gram stain on gastric aspirate; 3. depression of the infant's polymorph count to less than $2500/mm^3$; or 4. pyrexia in the infant or patchy chest X-ray changes.

If any of these features are present, then antibiotics, usually a penicillin and aminoglycoside must be given; conversely the absence of these features does not *exclude* pneumonia, and for this reason we put all dyspnoeic newborn infants on antibiotics until cultures are known to be negative.

Congenital malformations
Many malformations can cause dyspnoea in the first few hours of life (Table 5.5). Some are fatal, others require urgent transfer for surgical correction.

Table 5.5 Congenital malformations causing neonatal respiratory difficulty.

Congenital anomalies of the bony thorax
Diaphragmatic hernia
Chylothorax
Congenital lobar emphysema
Pulmonary agenesis
Pulmonary hypoplasia — Potter's syndrome
Congenital cystic adenomatoid malformation
Tracheal abnormalities — (stenosis, agenesis)
Upper airways obstruction (choanal atresia, Pierre–Robin syndrome)
Tracheo-oesophageal fistula
All causes of hydrops and pleural effusion

Chronic lung problems in very low birthweight (VLBW) infants

Recurrent Apnoea
Infants weighing less than 1.50 kg commonly develop episodes of apnoea which may last long enough for cyanosis and bradycardia to occur. Recurrent

Table 5.6 Causes of neonatal apnoea. From *A Manual of Neonatal Intensive Care* by Roberton, N.R.C. (1981). Edward Arnold, London.

RDS — deteriorating or undiagnosed
Massive pulmonary haemorrhage
Other lung disease eg. Wilson-Mikity pneumorthorax
Septicaemia, meningitis, pneumonia
Hypocalcaemia
Hypoglycaemia
Heart failure — especially pulmonary oedema with a persistent ductus arteriosis
Intracranial haemorrhage especially intraventricular haemorrhage
Convulsions
Respiratory depression by drugs
Aspiration and inhalation of a feed
Rare metabolic disease — consider only if the infant has other appropriate signs.

---

apnoea of this type may indicate serious underlying disease (Table 5.6) but, in infants in whom these diagnoses can be excluded, the apnoea usually represents immaturity of the central control of respiration. In such infants, most of the apnoeic attacks can be prevented by treatment with oral theophylline. Rarely the attacks are so severe and prolonged that assisted ventilation is necessary.

Treatment of an apnoeic attack
A peripheral stimulus is usually all that is required to make an apnoeic infant cry and start to breathe. Great care should always be taken in these infants, who are very susceptible to retrolental fibroplasia, to prevent surges in PaO_2 during resuscitation. If such an infant needs assisted ventilation, this should be given with the gas mixture which he is normally breathing. *NEVER* treat an apnoeic attack by giving the infant oxygen to breathe by face mask.

Wilson–Mikity syndrome
This usually occurs in VLBW infants who have not previously suffered from RDS. It presents at the age of 2–3 weeks with increasing dyspnoea and increased oxygen requirements; the aetiology is uncertain, but the chest X-ray shows predominantly upper lobe 'honeycomb' shadowing. In most infants the disease runs a benign course, though supplementary oxygen may be required for 6–8 weeks. Great care should be taken to avoid giving too much oxgyen, as these infants are at risk of retrolental fibroplasia.

Bronchopulmonary dysplasia
This is the lung fibrosis that results from long-term high pressure IPPV for RDS. Severe cases die without coming off the ventilator, and less severely affected babies may remain breathless and oxygen-dependent for some months. Severe cases may be helped by regular diuretic therapy.

Cardiac problems in the neonate

Neonatal heart disease usually presents in one of three ways; cyanosis, heart failure, or asymptomatic murmur.

Table 5.7 Differential diagnosis of cyanotic congenital heart disease. From Pickering. D., in: *A Manual of Neonatal Intensive Care* by Roberton, N.R.C. (1981). Edward Arnold, London.

Differential diagnosis of cardiac causes of neonatal cyanosis	Physiological arrangement	S₂P	ECG	CTR	MPA	VAS	Chest x-ray
Transitional circulation (1/1400 deliveries)	Block + hole	+	RAD ≫ RVH	N/+	N	N	May have aspiration features
Total pulmonary atresia or severe pulmonary stenosis with intact intraventricular septum (7.6%)*	Block + hole	–	RAH, LVH	N/+	–	–	Normal or enlarged heart, Decreased vascularity. No PA.
Tricuspid atresia (21%)*	Block + hole	–	LAD, LVH, RAH	N	–	–	'Square' heart ± enlarged. Decreased vascularity. No PA. Prominent SVC.
Tricuspid incompetence caused by Ebsteins (0.32%)*	Block + hole	+	PRBB, WPW, RAH	+	–	–	Improves spontaneously.
Total anomalous venous drainage (obstructed type)	Scrambled veins	+	RAD, RAH, marked RVH	N	+	+	Small heart with no pulmonary venous congestion.
Transposition of great arteries (17.4%)*	Scrambled arteries	+	Normal or RAD, RVH	+	–	N/+	Narrow base frontal compared with wide base RAO. 25% 'egg'-shaped heart on narrow pedicle.
Tetralogy (7.1%) and tetralogy-like lesions	Block + hole	–	RAD, RVH	N	–	–	'Boot'-shaped heart.
Truncus arteriosus (1.7%)	Common mixing	+	RVH, LVH	+	–	+	'Long-toed' boot with increased vascularity but no PA.

S₂P Intensity of second sound in pulmonary area; CTR, Cardiothoracic ratio; MPA, Size of the main pulmonary artery on radiograph; SVC, (Superior vena cava); RAD, Right axis deviation; N, Normal; LAD, Left axis deviation; LVH, Left ventricular hypertrophy; PRBB, Partial right bundle branch block; WPW, Wolffe Parkinson White; RAH, Right atrial hypertrophy; RAO, Right anterior oblique projection at radiograph; RHV, Right ventricular hypertrophy; PA, Pulmonary artery; VAS, Vascularity.
*Figures in brackets indicate incidence of cardiac malformations in the first month of life from the data of Keith, Rowe and Vlad (1978).

Cyanotic heart disease

Infants with malformations causing cyanotic congenital heart disease usually present in the first 2–3 days of life. In addition to the cyanosis they have difficulty in feeding and dyspnoea due to pulmonary oedema. However, infants with uncorrectable malformations may remain surprisingly asymptomatic and pink for several days after delivery.

On examination subtle abnormalities of the heart sounds, or a very soft murmur may be all that there is to detect, though there may be hepatosplenomegaly from congestive cardiac failure. The ECG and chest X-ray are usually abnormal; arterial blood gas analysis shows a normal to low CO_2, commonly some degree of metabolic acidosis, and a PO_2 in the range 3.5–5.5 kPa (25–44 mmHg) which changes very little when the infant breathes 100 per cent oxygen. The differential diagnosis of the various types of cyanotic heart disease is given in Table 5.7. Echo-cardiography is extremely useful in such infants, since if the gross cardiac anatomy is normal then the likely diagnosis is either lung disease or persistence of the fetal circulation. However a definitive diagnosis requires referral to a regional cardiac centre.

Persistence of the fetal circulation is the likely diagnosis if the chest X-ray and ECG are within normal limits or only mildly abnormal. Cardiac catheterization shows the pulmonary blood pressure is at systemic level with a patent ductus and a patent foramen ovale (i.e. a fetal circulatory pattern). If persistence of the fetal circulation is suspected the appropriate treatment is to give intravenous tolazoline (a pulmonary vasodilator) or to hyperventilate the neonate to $PaCO_2$ of 25 mmHg, which also dilates the pulmonary arteries.

Table 5.8 Causes of cardiac failure in early infancy. From Pickering, D., in: *A Manual of Neonatal Intensive Care* by Roberton, N.R.C. (1981). Edward Arnold, London.

Premature infants:
    Persistent ductus arteriosus (PDA)
    Ventricular septal defects (VSD)
    Metabolic — hypocalcaemia, hypomagnesaemia, hypoglycaemia, poycythaemia,
        acidaemia, hypoxia
    Combined defects — PDA plus hypoxia, VSD and PDA

Birth to one week (left ventricular failure occurs more often than right ventricular failure):
    Hypoplastic left heart
    Coarctation of the aorta syndrome
    Aortic stenosis
    Transient myocardial ischaemia in the newborn
    Interrupted aortic arch
    Cardiomyopathies — Coxsackie myocarditis type B
    Rhythm disturbances — paroxsymal supraventricular tachycardia
    Arterioventricular or semilunar valve incompetence
    Arteriovenous fistulae — cerebral or hepatic

One week to one month:
    VSD
    PDA
    Truncus arteriosus
    Total anomalous pulmonary venous drainage (non-obstructive type)
    Endocardial cushion defect

The neonate in congestive cardiac failure

Heart failure causes tachypnoea of greater than 50–60/min and a tachycardia often with a gallop rhythm. The babies are often pale and sweaty. Pulmonary crepitations are heard and hepatosplenomegaly develops; periphral oedema is rare.

Causes of congestive cardiac failure in the first week are very different from those seen later in life (Table 5.8); the diagnosis can often be made from the history alone. If further investigation is needed it should include an ECG and chest X-ray plus appropriate tests to exclude the various metabolic, infective and toxic causes. If there are murmurs or abnormal heart sounds, and structural abnormalities are suspected, echocardiography is an essential component of the workup.

Congestive cardiac failure should be treated with fluid restriction, diuretics and digoxin, and in most cases the infant's condition will improve. If it does not, and a structural problem is responsible, early referral to a regional cardiac centre is necessary. If a low output state is responsible for the heart failure, plasma expanders and the use of inotropic drugs such as dopamine are often necessary.

Patent ductus arteriosus
This occurs in up to 50 per cent of VLBW infants who need IPPV for RDS. It usually presents at the end of the first week of life, the infant developing signs of heart failure plus bounding pulses and a systolic murmur heard maximally in the pulmonary area. As well as controlling heart failure the oral administration of a prostaglandin synthetase inhibitor such as indomethacin will close the PDA.

The asymptomatic murmur

The vast majority of murmurs heard in otherwise asymptomatic neonates are systolic and will disappear. The earlier in life these are heard, the more likely this it to be true, since many infants have short midsystolic noises in the first 24–48 hours of life as the heart converts to the adult circulatory pattern.

Even when these murmurs are heard at the age of 7 days they are likely to disappear, since they often arise from small shunts through a patent ductus or ventricular septal defect which will close in the subsequent weeks and months. However in such infants the femoral pulses must always be carefully checked, and signs of congestive cardiac failure excluded. It is prudent in most cases to check the chest X-ray and ECG prior to discharge from the maternity hospital and to ensure that the baby is followed up.

Infection in the neonate

There is no IgA or IgM in the plasma of newborn infants, and preterm infants have very low levels of IgG, unlike full-term infants who have normal levels of this immunoglobulin acquired transplacentally from their mothers. Full-term neonates have low complement levels and diminished polymorphonuclear and lymphocyte function compared with older children, with these deficiences more marked in the premature infant.

As a result, neonates are not only more prone to infection but infection once established disseminates extemely rapidly. The most common organisms responsible for serious infection in the neonate are; *E. coli*, group B *streptococcus*, *Staphylococcus aureus*, other gram negative *bacilli-proteus-klebsiella*, *pseudomonas*, and *Listeria monocytogenes*.

However most organisms, including viruses and anaerobes, can cause overwhelming neonatal infection.

Signs and symptoms

It is essential to have a very low threshold of suspicion for infection in neonates, and every effort must be made to establish the diagnosis on the basis of early and subtle clinical signs:

1. Pallor, skin mottling, restlessness and hypotonia.
2. Anorexia, mild diarrhoea and vomiting.
3. Temperature increase or decrease.
4. Jaundice.
5. Recurrent apnoea or tachypnoea.
6. Irritability.
7. Pseudoparalysis (indicating arthritis or ostemyelitis).
8. Ileus, abdominal distension.

Cyanosis, cough and overt respiratory difficutly are late signs of pneumonia; while neck retraction, a bulging fontanelle and seizures are late signs of meningitis. Both these conditions should be diagnosed on the basis of the more subtle clinical signs outlined above, before more florid symptoms develop.

A full clinical examination should always be carried out in an infant suspected of infection, although, apart from confirming the presenting signs, other physical signs are rare.

Diagnosis and treatment

All infants suspected of infection should have the following investigation:

1. Swabs from all lesions, also from the nose, throat and umbilical stump.
2. Bag urine analysis.
3. Blood culture.
4. White count and differential; this is a good screening test; less than 2.5×10^9/litre or more than 8.0×10^9/litre polymorphs/mm^3 is very suggestive of infection in the neonate.
5. Chest X-ray.
6. Lumbar puncture (in most cases).

Since it is essential not to miss the diagnosis of infection in infants, unless there are good reasons for procrastinating, antibiotics should be started as soon as the investigations listed above have been carried out. The antibiotics of choice will vary from hospital to hospital, but in general the combination of a penicillin and an aminoglycoside is given — say penicillin G plus gentamicin; until the results of cultures are known. If these are all negative, and the infant's symptoms rapidly settle, the antibiotics can be stopped after 2–3 days. However if infection is confirmed, antibiotics should be given for 10 days, continuing for 14 days in the case of septicaemia and even longer in meningitis. In infants with meningitis due to Gram negative organisms, intrathecal and intraventricular therapy are usually required.

Necrotizing enterocolitis
This is a complex disease (Fig. 5.5). Gut ischaemia and fluid overload have occurred in most cases. The infant has usually been milk fed, and gut infection with coliforms, anaerobes or clostridia is also important and may be the sole cause in some cases.

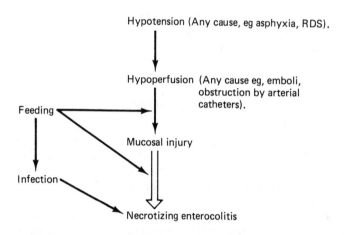

Fig. 5.5   Aetiological factors in necrotizing enterocolitis.

Necrotizing enterocolitis presents with the signs of infection (p. 61) plus abdominal distension and bloody stools; paralytic ileus and ascites develop in many cases. Abdominal X-ray shows an oedematous gut wall with intramural gas, and in some cases free intraperitoneal air indicating gut perforation. Treatment is to stop all oral feeds and to aspirate the infant's stomach 4 hourly through a naso-gastric tube and maintain hydration intravenously for at least one week. These patients require routine intensive care with maintenance of acid–base and electrolyte homeostasis plus frequent blood and plasma transfusions; nutrition is given parenterally. If gut perforation occurs most surgeons would recommend laparotomy and resection of the necrotic bowel. The overall mortality remains 20–30 per cent.

Superficial infections
If the care of the umbilical stump is satisfactory (p. 33) superficial infections are rare. If periumbilical redness develops, usually caused by staphylococci or *E.coli*, swabs should be taken and the stump sprayed with an antibiotic powder. Occasionally superficial staphylococcal skin infections occur in infants but this can be treated with oral flucloxacillin. Thrush, which is usually a trivial oral or perianal infection in the neonate, should be treated with topical nystatin. The treatment of conjunctivitis is given in Table 5.9.

Table 5.9 Differential diagnosis and treatment of neonatal conjuctivitis. From *A Manual of Neonatal Intensive Care* by Roberton, N.R.C. (1981). Edward Arnold, London

Organism	Age at presentation	Diagnosis	Treatment
N. gonorrhoeae	1 day (more now recognized later in 1st week)	Maternal history – promiscuity etc.	Intramuscular penicillin
		Profuse conjunctival discharge	Penicillin eye drops hourly
		Urgent Gram-stain on pus shows Gram – ve intracellular diplococci	Notifiable disease, Remember to treat mother and consorts
		Culture of swab sent in transport medium	
Staph. aureus, Esch. coli	3–5 days peak, but may be at any time including day 1	Culture of swab	If mild: sterile saline cleaning
			If severe: 0.5% chloramphenicol eye drops
Chlamydia trachomatis	7 days	Venereal disease, therefore similar maternal history of gonorrhoeae	Chlortetracycline eye ointment + systemic erythromycin (30 mg/kg – for at least 2 weeks)
		Conventional cultures sterile. Chlamydial cultures positive	
		Positive conjunctival scraping for inclusion bodies	

Jaundice

Neonatal jaundice is virtually always an unconjugated hyperbilirubinaemia. This is unfortunate, since high levels of *free* bilirubin, which is present in nanomole quantities only and is the component of unconjugated bilirubin not bound to plasma albumin, is probably the compound which damages brain cells and causes kernicterus. Kernicterus may be fatal or cause severe mental subnormality, athetoid cerebral palsy or deafness in survivors. The level of free bilirubin at which kernicterus occurs is not known, but it probably rises to toxic levels when the *total* unconjugated bilirubin reaches 350 mmol/litre. However, mature and otherwise healthy infants do not develop kernicterus unless the total unconjugated bilirubin is much higher than 350 mmol/litre, whereas small sick preterm infants may devlop kernicterus at total unconjugated bilirubin levels around 200 mmol/litre.

Patterns of neonatal jaundice (Fig. 5.6)

Physiological
This is seen in 20–30 per cent of all full term infants, but is more common in

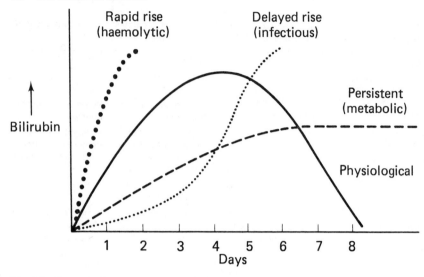

Fig. 5.6   Patterns of neonatal jaundice. (Reproduced from *A Manual of Neonatal Intensive Care* by Roberton, N.R.C. (1981). Edward Arnold, London.)

preterm infants. It rises to a peak, rarely greater than 250 mmol/litre on the 4th–6th day, and fades thereafter.

Factors which increase the likelihood of physiological jaundice are:

1. Immaturity of the liver enzymes which conjugate bilirubin to bilirubin glucuronide.
2. Shortened neonatal RBC survival.
3. Dehydration and starvation.
4. Bruising during delivery.
5. High haematocrit from delayed cord clamping.
6. Induction of delivery in the mother. Effect of the drugs?

If jaundice exceeds 250 mmol/litre after the third day, other diagnoses such as mild infection or haemolysis should be excluded, before a diagnosis of physiological jaundice is accepted. However, kernicterus is extraordinarily rare in infants with physiological jaundice alone, and the only treatment required even if the bilirubin exceeds 320 mmol/litre, is maintenance of fluid intake and occasionally phototherapy (p. 66). In term infants, exchange transfusion should only be considered if the total unconjugated bilirubin exceeds 400–425 mmol/litre.

Infectious jaundice
Jaundice which develops suddenly in any infant supports the diagnosis of infection, and appropriate investigations and treatment should be instituted (p. 61).

Haemolytic jaundice; haemolytic disease of the newborn
This should be the working diagnosis in all infants who become overtly jaundiced within 24 hours of delivery. In a few infants, haemolysis is due to an

inherent RBC defect such as spherocytosis or glucose-6-diphosphate deficiency, but much more commonly it is due to blood group incompatibility. In the 1980s, with the relative rarity of rhesus (D) incompatibility, ABO incompatibility, usually with a group O mother and a group A baby, is numerically much more important. Occasional cases of haemolytic disease of the newborn are seen due to other blood group antigens including other rhesus groups.

Infants with rhesus (D) incompatibility may be very anaemic at birth, with hepatosplenomegaly, and occasionally hypoproteinaemia, severe heart failure and peripheral oedema (hydrops fetalis); while infants with the other blood group incompatibilities usually present with rapid onset of jaundice alone.

In cases of rhesus incompatibility the diagnosis, and the severity of the disease are established in the antenatal period (p. 124). At delivery cord blood should be taken from all affected babies for haemoglobin, blood group, bilirubin and Coombs' test to confirm the diagnosis and estimate the severity of the disease. Infants with a cord blood haemoglobin less than 10 g/dl need urgent exchange transfusions to raise their haemoglobin and wash out antibody, and those with haemoglobin values of 10–14 g/dl will almost certainly need an exchange transfusion within the first 24 hours of life. Subsequent exchange transfusions in infants with rhesus (D) incompatibility are carried out to keep the serum bilirubin less than 350 mmol/litre. Phototherapy (p. 66) should also be given.

Similar investigations should also be carried out on the cord blood of all other neonates in whom haemolytic disease is suspected. In ABO incompatibility the Coombs' test is often negative, and the diagnosis is based on the appropriate blood group set up and the presence of anti-A haemolysin in the mother's serum. In these infants, as in those with other nonrhesus haemolytic disease, urgent exchange transfusion is rarely required, and in most cases the jaundice can be controlled with phototherapy. However if the bilirubin exceeds 350 mmol/litre exchange transfusion is indicated.

Persisting jaundice

There are many causes (Table 5.10) and specific investigation should always be carried out in an infant who is still jaundiced at 2–3 weeks of age, particularly to exclude galactosaemia and cretinism, treatable causes of mental retardation.

Investigation of neonatal jaundice

The tests to be done in jaundiced infants presenting at different ages are shown in Table 5.11.

Treatment

Exchange transfusion is required in infants at risk of kernicterus. Successive 10–20 ml aliquots of the infant's blood are removed by syringe from a central catheter, and then replaced with 10–20 ml aliquots of fresh (less than 2-day-old) bank blood stored in citrate-phosphate-dextrose. A total of 160 ml/kg body weight is usually exchanged.

Table 5.10 Causes of prolonged neonatal jaundice. From *A Manual of Neonatal Intensive Care* by Roberton, N.R.C. (1981). Edward Arnold, London

---

Group I **Persistence of acute neonatal cause (unconjugated)**
    Haemolytic anaemia (immune, spherocytic or non-spherocytic)
    Chronic/low grade infection (bacterial or viral)

Group II **Rare (unconjugated)**
    Galactosaemia
    Hypothyroidism
    Aminoacidaemia (increased tyrosine, methionine)
    Breast feeding (conjugation inhibitors in milk)
    Drugs
    Lucey–Driscoll syndrome (serum conjugation inhibitor)
    Crigler–Najjar syndromes
    Cystic fibrosis
    Gilberts's disease

Group III **Obstructive jaundice**
    Hepatitis
        a) Congenital infection (rubella, cytomegalovirus etc.)
        b) Giant cell neonatal hepatitis
        c) Positive Australia antigen
        d) Galactosaemia
    Insipissated bile syndrome (post severe Rh haemolytic disease)
    Cystic fibrosis
    Biliary atresia
    α_1 antitrypsin deficiency
    Inherited defects (Dubin–Johnson, Rotor)
    Extrinsic biliary obstruction (band, tumour, cholodochal cyst)

Phototherapy

Light at the blue end of the spectrum (425–475 nm) photoisomerizes unconjugated bilirubin into a nontoxic, colourless, water soluble form. Phototherapy is indicated in infants in whom exchange transfusion might be necessary to prevent kernicterus. It is not necessary in term asymptomatic infants unless the bilirubin exceeds 320–350 mmol/litre.

Neurological problems in the neonate

Neonatal fits have many causes (Table 5.12). Although it is often possible, on the basis of the history and clinical examination, to make an educated guess in an individual baby, at the aetiology, all infants who have fits should have the following investigations carried out:

1. Blood glucose.
2. Serum electrolytes and blood urea.
3. Serum calcium.
4. WBC and differential.
5. Blood culture.
6. Lumbar puncture.
7. Cerebral ultrasound.

In a small number of infants it will still not be possible to establish a diagnosis. In most of these cases, only a few fits will occur, the infant will

Table 5.11 Investigation of neonatal jaundice. From *A Manual of Neonatal Intensive Care* by Roberton, N.R.C. (1981). Edward Arnold, London

Rapidly developing jaundice on the first day

	Diagnosis	Test
Likely	Rhesus, ABO and other haemolytic disease	Haemoglobin, direct Coombs' test, Group
	Spherocytosis	Blood film, check family history
Unlikely	Congenital infection	IgM, serology, platelet count, culture
	Non-spherocytic haemolytic anaemia including G6PD deficiency	Appropriate enzyme test May present later than 1st day

Rapid onset jaundice after the first 48 hours

	Diagnosis	Test
Likely	Infection	WBC, culture all sites, bag urine, blood culture, lumbar puncture, chest X ray
Unlikely	Conditions listed above detected late	See above

Persistent jaundice beyond 10 days

	Diagnosis	Test
Likely	Normal breast-fed infant	Observe if clinically well and gaining weight
	Persisting infection	As for infection above
Unlikely	Conditions in Tables 11.5 and 11.6: must exclude hepatitis, galactosaemia, hypothyroidism	Appropriate blood and urine tests

Jaundice greater than 250 mmol/litre (15 mg%) on day 3–5

Infant asymptomatic, feeding well, but yellow. Probably marked physiological jaundice. Nevertheless do the following tests.
Mid-stream urine for asymptomatic urinary infection.
White blood count for latent infection.
Group and direct Coombs' test for mild haemolytic disease of the newborn which could be significant in subsequent pregnancies.
Consider RBC enzyme studies in appropriate ethnic group.

---

remain neurologically normal, and the cause of the fits will never be established, though they are probably an aftermath of mild perinatal brain injury. Only if the fits persist or are difficult to control, is there the need to perform more complicated metabolic investigations, or to carry out an EEG or CT scan.

As well as treating any underlying cause, the fits should be stopped with intravenous diazepam or phenobarbitone and maintenance phenobarbitone therapy should be given in most cases.

Table 5.12 Differential diagnosis of causes of neonatal convulsions. From *A Manual of Neonatal Intensive Care* by Roberton, N.R.C. (1981). Edward Arnold, London

Diagnosis	Age at presentation and type of fit	Other factors
Birth asphyxia	0–72 hours, usually clonic, may be tonic/ apnoea	History of intrapartum asphyxia
With cerebral oedema	As above	As above + bulging, tense fontanelle, head retraction
With subarachnoid or subdural haemorrhage	As above	As above + blood on lumbar puncture
Intraventricular haemorrhage	24-72 hours, usually tonic	Rare > 1.50 kg: often in infants with severe RDS or recurrent apnoea. Decreased packed cell volume. Lumbar puncture blood stained. Blood in ventricles on ventricular puncture or ultrasound
Hypoxia	Any time and any type of fit — usually 0-72 hours	in a very sick infant — especially post-episodes of respiratory or cardiac arrest
Meningitis	Any time any type of fit	Associated signs of sepsis: lumbar puncture
Metabolic Hypoglycaemia	Usually <48 hours and clonic	Small-for-date infant, prem. baby. If later, suggests rare causes of hypoglycaemia
Hypocalcaemia	<48 hours tonic or clonic: 5–8 days; multifocal clonic	Usually seriously ill infant High phosphate intake
Hypomagnesaemia	5–8 days; multi-focal clonic	Usually with hypocalcaemia
Hyponatraemia	Any age; usually clonic	Usually an oedematous sick preterm infant.
Hypernatraemia	Any age; usually clonic	Usually sick, underhydrated preterm infant.
Rare inborn errors of metabolism	Usually <72 hours; any type of fit	Often apnoeic, hypotonic, positive family history
Kernicterus	Any time, any type of fit	Associated with severe jaundice
Congenital malformation or infection	Any time, any type of fit	Other physical signs and stigmata
Drug withdrawal	Usually <1 week; usually clonic	Mother's drug history
Idopathic	Any time, usually clonic	By exclusion

Intracranial haemorrhage

Neonatal subdural haemorrhage is rare and virtually always associated with severe and fatal birth asphyxia. Subarachnoid haemorrhage is probably comparatively common, rarely causing problems other than seizures (see above).

The most important form of neonatal cerebral haemorrhage is intraventricular haemorrhage (IVH), which is now the commonest cause of death in very low birthweight infants and is particularly common in those suffering from RDS. An IVH arises at the anterior end of the floor of the lateral ventricle, between the ependyma and the caudate nucleus. It may be confined in that layer when it is known as germinal layer haemorrhage, or it may rupture through the ependyma into the ventricular system becoming an IVH.

IVH is comparatively rare in infants greater than 1.50 kg birthweight, but may occur in 50 per cent of infants weighing less than this. A small IVH is often asymptomatic, but a large IVH normally causes the infant to collapse with apnoea, hypotonia, multiple seizures and coma; rapidly progressing to death.

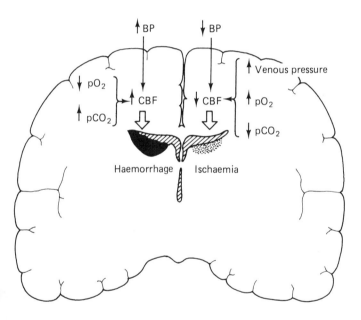

Fig. 5.7 Aetiology of intraventricular haemorrhage (IVH). (With permission from Wigglesworth, J.S. (1978). *Early Human Development* **2**, 179–99.)

The aetiology of IVH is summarized in Fig. 5.7. The capillaries in the germinal layer are very fragile, and become even more fragile if the area becomes ischemic during episodes of hypotension or some other cause of reduced cerebral blood flow (CBF). Anything that subsequently causes a rise in CBF (e.g. a decrease in PaO_2 or an increase in $PaCO_2$), or a surge in systolic BP (since CBF in sick preterm infants does not autoregulate) will cause a torrential flow through these capillaries which may rupture, causing the germinal layer or intraventricular haemorrhage.

Treatment

A large IVH is fatal, but after a small bleed the infant can survive if blood gas and electrolyte homeostasis are maintained, and blood volume and pressure are kept normal. Such infants may subsequently need treatment for hydrocephalus if the haemorrhage impedes the cerebrospinal fluid circulation.

Abnormalities of tone

The clinical significance of abnormalities of tone, in the absence of an abnormal history or other physical signs suggestive of CNS disease can be exaggerated. Marked hypertonia plus jitteryness should be assessed in the same way as infants with seizures, and if marked hypotonia persists the conditions listed in Table 5.13 should be excluded.

Table 5.13 Causes of hypotonia in a neonate.

Drug depression
Septicaemia
Asphyxial brain damage
Hypoglycaemia
Prematurity
Rarities: Spinal cord injuries
Werdnig–Hoffman disease
Myasthenia
Myotonic dystrophy
Congenital myopathies
Inborn error of metabolism
Benign congenital hypotonia

Metabolic problems

Hypoglycaemia

Normal full-term, preterm and small-for-dates infants have blood glucose values in the range 1.5–3.5 mmol/litre in the first few days of life; levels which would cause symptoms of neuroglycopenia in older children and adults. By definition, hypoglycaemia in the neonate is said to occur when the blood glucose is less than 1.0 mmol/litre, and is seen primarily in small-for-dates infants and sick VLBW infants.

Surprisingly, even infants with blood glucose levels below 1.0 mmol/litre may remain asymptomatic for several hours before they develop the only significant symptoms of hypoglycaemia; apnoea or fits.

Hypoglycaemia, symptomatic or otherwise is preventable in most neonates by adequate oral feeding or intravenous 5–10 per cent glucose. However, small-for-dates and sick VLBW infants must be screened by dextrostix 4–8 hourly during the first 48–72 hours of life, to ensure that blood glucose levels falling below 1.0 mmol/litre are detected while the infant is still asymptomatic. If asymptomatic hypoglycaemia is detected in an infant who is being fed, the appropriate therapy is to give another milk feed, progressing to IV glucose if the blood glucose does not rise above 1.0 mmol/litre following the feed. If symptomatic hypoglycaemia occurs in any infant he should be given 10 ml of 10 per cent glucose intravenously at once, followed by an infusion of 10 per cent glucose at the appropriate rate for his body weight.

Infants of diabetic mothers

Infants of inadequately controlled diabetic mothers are hyperinsulinaemic immediately after delivery, and may become profoundly hypoglycaemic (less than 0.5 mmol/litre) by 1–2 hours of age. This virtually always recovers spontaneously by 3–4 hours of age and the infant remains asymptomatic, comes to no harm, and requires no treatment. If the hypoglycaemia persists, or if other symptoms develop, an intravenous infusion of dextrose should be set up and maintained with great care to prevent rebound hypoglycaemia.

Infants of diabetic mothers have an increased incidence of jaundice, RDS, hypocalcaemia and congenital malformation.

Electrolyte disturbances

Sick neonates are prone to hypernatraemia, hyponatraemia, hyperkalaemia, hypokalaemia and commonly hypocalcaemia. These can usually be controlled by daily measurement of plasma electrolytes, plus meticulous attention to fluid and electrolyte balance, giving appropriate infusions of each cation to the babies.

Haematological problems

Haemorrhagic disease of the newborn

Newborn infants, particularly those born prematurely, may bleed from the gut, cord stump or incisions (e.g. circumcision) on the second to fourth day of life, due to deficiency of the vitamin K dependent factors (II, VIII, IX, X). This condition must be prevented by giving 1 mg of vitamin K (Konakion) intramuscularly to every newborn baby.

Anaemia

Pallor in the neonate can be due to asphyxia or sepsis as well as anaemia. Anaemia immediately after delivery may be due to rhesus haemolytic disease or may be the result of a fetal bleed during the second stage of labour, or a feto–maternal or twin to twin haemorrhage at any time before labour. A haemoglobin less than 8–10 g/dl irrespective of its cause in the first few hours or days of life, particularly if accompanied by symptoms such as dyspnoea or hypotension, needs urgent treatment by a top up or exchange transfusion.

Anaemia detected at any stage in the neonatal period in asymptomatic infants can be more carefully investigated, and the transfusion only given if the haemoglobin is less than 8 g/dl and causes dyspnoea or difficulty feeding, and seems unlikely to rise spontaneously.

Congenital malformations

This is an enormous topic, and in this section only a brief synopsis will be given of some of those malformations which cause problems in the neonatal period.

Intestinal abnormalities

Tracheo-oesophageal fistula
In 90 per cent of the cases this is the coexistence of upper oesophageal atresia, with a fistula from the carina to the lower oesophageal remnant. It presents within the first hours of life with pooling of secretions in the oesphageal stump followed by aspiration. Failure to pass a nasogastric tube and demonstrating that the tube is curled up in the proximal oesphageal pouch on plain X-ray confirms the diagnosis. Treatment is surgical with anastomosis of the proximal and distal oesophageal segments, plus division of the fistula.

Diaphragmatic hernia
This usually presents as severe neonatal respiratory difficulty and the diagnosis is made on the chest X-ray (p. 51). Urgent surgical repair is required, but the mortality is high due to associated severe pulmonary hypoplasia.

Neonatal gut obstruction
This usually presents with abdominal distension, failure to pass meconium and a bile stained gastric aspirate. The causes and differential diagnosis are given in Table 5.14. Those due to structural obstruction, as opposed to necrotizing enterocolitis or paralytic ileus, require urgent surgery.

Table 5.14 Differential diagnosis of abdominal distension and bilious vomiting in the neonate

Condition	Evaluation and differential diagnosis
Necrotising enterocolitis	Generally septic picture and blood in stools; abdominal X-ray; fluid levels, gas in bowel wall and ascites (p. 62)
Paralytic ileus	Any very sick infant e.g. RDS, severe haemolytic disease of the newborn or electrolyte imbalance
Small intestinal atresia including postampullary duodenal atresia and volvulus with malrotation	Infant otherwise well. Plain X-ray; fluid levels, though infant may have passed meconium; Barium meal usually establishes the diagnosis
Meconium ileus	Family history of cystic fibrosis; peculiar bubbly gut contents on abdominal X-ray; infants rarely pass meconium

Abnormalities of the genito-urinary tract

Potter's Syndrome
This common anomaly comprises multiple postural abnormalities as a result

of oligohydramnios, plus pulmonary hypoplasia and renal agenesis. The infants are very small-for-dates and present at birth with severe respiratory distress due to the lung lesion. The condition is fatal.

Malformations
Posterior urethral valves, hydronephrosis and cystic kidneys present in the neonatal period with bladder enlargement and dribbling micturition in the former, and flank masses in the latter two. Appropriate investigation by ultrasound and contrast radiography must be carried out, and the first two conditions require urgent surgery.

Intersex
The infant presenting with ambiguous genitalia is commonly a female infant virilized by congenital adrenal hyperplasia. This diagnosis can be confirmed by measuring an increased level of 17-hydroxyprogesterone in the plasma. Other causes of ambiguous genitalia are given in Table 5.15. These require urgent evaluation by cytogenetic, radiological and endocrinological means.

Table 5.15 Causes of ambiguous genitalia in the neonate. From *A Manual of Neonatal Intensive Care* by Roberton, N.R.C. (1981). Edward Arnold, London.

Female pseudohermaphroditism:
    maternal androgen/progestorone therapy
    Congenital adrenal hyperplasia

Male pseudohermaphroditism:
    Extreme perineoscrotal hypospadias
    Endocrine causes (testosterone biosynthetic defects)
    Testicular feminization syndrome
    Rare variants of congenital adrenal hyperplasia (CAH)

Genetic defects:
    Turner's syndrome
    Mosaics of similar chromosomal constitution
    True hermaphrodites

Neural tube malformations

Anencephalus is universally fatal and small closed meningoceles do not require urgent therapy and will not be considered here.

Table 5.16 Adverse clinical features in a neonate with myelomeningocele. From *A Manual of Neonatal Intensive Care* by Roberton, N.R.C. (1981). Edward Arnold, London.

Total paraplegia or minimal hip flexion only

Kyphoscoliosis present at birth

Hydrocephalus (occipitofrontal circumference) at least 2 cm >90th centile for gestation

A large thoracolumbar lesion (>four spinal segements)

Associated malformations (congenital heart disease)

Table 5.17 Clinical features of autosomal trisomies diagnosable at birth. From *A Manual of Neonatal Intensive Care* by Roberton, N.R.C. (1981), Edward Arnold, London.

	Trisomy 21 Mongolism— Down's syndrome	Trisomy 18 Edward's syndrome	Trisomy 13 Patau's syndrome
Incidence	1:600	1:2000	1:5000
General	Happy, docile children. Enjoy mimicry and listening to music Small for dates	Feeble cry, premature or postmature Small for dates	Small for dates
Growth	Slower than normal	Survival rare	Survival rare
CNS	Hypotonia, IQ 25–50	Hypertonic IQ retarded	Holoprosencephaly; agenesis of corpus callosum, spina bifida, hypertonic IQ decreased
Cranium	Flat occiput, 3rd fontanelle microcephaly	Prominent occiput, narrow bifrontal diameter, microcephaly	Wide fontanelle, hyperterlorism, microcephaly
Eyes	Upward slanting eyes, squint; epicanthus, Brushfield's spots	Short palpebral fissure, epicanthus	Micro-opthalmia, coloboma anophthalmia, cyclopia
Ears	Small overlapping helices, low set	Low set and malformed	Low set, odd helices, deaf
Nose	Small, low nasal bridge	—	—
Mouth	Small maxilla and palate; fissured, protruding tongue	Small, narrow, arched palate, micrognathia, cleft lip and palate	Hare lip, cleft palate, cleft tongue, micrognathia
Neck	Broad, short	—	—
Chest	—	Abnormal or absent right lung, short sternum, hypoplastic nipples	—
Hands	Short hands and fingers, single palmar crease, clinodactyly of 5th fingers, distal palmar triradius	Clenched with overlapping finger, small nails, ulnar deflection of hand, small thumb	Overlapping fingers, distal triradius, hyperconvex nails, polydactyly, ulnar deflection, radial aplasia, syndactyly
Feet	Gap between 1st and 2nd toes	Small hallux, talipes equinovarus, rocker bottom feet	Rocker bottom, small nails, and talipes equinovarus
Gut and abdomen	Diastasis recti, duodenal atresia, tracheo-oesophageal, fistula, Hirschprung's disease	Umbilical hernia, malformation of anus, Meckel's divarticulum	Omphalocele, umbilical hernia, malrotation
Skin	Dry	Redundant and hairy	Haemangiomata, scalp defects, loose neck skin
Cardiovascular	atrioventricular valve canal, ventricular septal defects	ventricular septal defects, arterial septal defects	ventricular septal defects, patent ductus arteriosus, dextrocardia
Genitalla/	—	Hydronephrosis, polycystic kidneys, cryptorchid, small labia, horseshoe kidney	Cryptorchid, odd scrotum bicornumia, uterus hypospadias, polycystic kidneys, hydronephrosis
X-ray	Hypoplastic acetabula and flat acetabular and iliac angles, hypoplastic mid phalanx 5th finger	—	Pelvic hypoplasia, thin ribs

Open myelomeningocele

Babies born with this lesion require careful clinical assessment by an experienced paediatrician and neurosurgeon, combined with radiological and ultrasound examination. There must also be discussion with the parents' GP, and of course several with the parents themselves. In general infants with major problems, such as those outlined in Table 5.16 should not be operated on in the early neonatal period. They should have their lesion cleaned, and be fed on demand and be allowed home if that is their parents' wish. If major problems are absent, the spinal defect should be closed to prevent subarachnoid infection. Treatment of the hydrocephalus, orthopaedic and surgical problems can be planned subsequently.

Chromosomal anomalies and dysmorphic infants

Sex chromosomes aneuploidy is rarely recognisable in the neonatal period, but the autosomal trisomies are. Their clinical features are given in Table 5.17. Trisomy 13 and 18 are rapidly fatal conditions. With all other malformed infants, chromosome analysis should always be carried out, and the infant's dysmorphic features checked in the many atlases of these syndromes which are now available (e.g. Smith 1982).

Further reading

Roberton, N.R.C. (1981). *A Manual of Neonatal Intensive Care.* Edward Arnold (Publishers), London.
Smith, D.W. (1982). *Recognizable Patterns of Human Malformation*, 3rd Edition. W.B. Saunders, London and Toronto.

6

The puerperium

This is the time taken to recover from pregnancy and delivery. It starts after completion of the third stage and includes the initial ten day period during which the mother and the baby are usually cared for by a midwife. For practical purposes the puerperium ends when the mother has her postnatal examination, usually about 6 weeks after delivery. The process of recovery, however, varies according to the woman's health after delivery and whether she suffers any complications. As she has to look after her new baby, this is a time of hard work rather than convalescence; there are disturbed nights, anxieties over coping with the baby and its progress as well as commitments to husband, home and other children. Breast-feeding is a drain, albeit physiological, on the physical resources of the mother. In physiological terms, the return to normal may take a period of months and cannot be completed until breast-feeding has stopped.

Care in the days immediately following delivery

The patient may leave hospital on the day of delivery, though this is not a very widespread practice at present, or any time during the ten days after delivery. In Britain she remains under the care of a registered midwife, whether at home or in hospital during this time.

Observations

General
The general condition and appearance of the woman should be noted first. She may be fit and happy, ill, anxious, depressed or tired and sleeping badly.

Specific Observations
The temperature and pulse should be recorded daily, the level of the uterine fundus measured and recorded (it is helpful to do this when the bladder is empty since a full bladder displaces the uterus upwards).

The Uterus should feel hard and the fundus will be palpable approximately at the level of the umbilicus on the first day; it should be lower day by day, reaching the midpoint between the tenth and the fourteenth day. The patient may suffer 'after pains', painful contractions of the uterus which are particularly likely to occur while the infant is feeding at the breast. They are not abnormal, but may be severe enough for the woman to require an analgesic.

Discharge There is a discharge from the uterus, the lochia. Initially this is quite heavy and contains mainly blood, red at first but gradually becoming darker. After 7–10 days the amount of blood should be small and the discharge may be clear or yellow, but it is not uncommon to find that women have continued to lose blood until shortly before they come for their postnatal examination. The lochia should not be offensive, and if it is there is likely to be a genital tract infection, while a heavy loss suggests retained products of conception. (See p. 94)

Perineal Repair Any perineal repair should be checked to ensure that there is no dehiscence or infection. If the perineum is particularly painful it should be checked to exclude a haematoma, and ice packs and analgesics used to relieve the discomfort. The use of rubber rings will reduce pressure on the area when seated. Nonabsorbable sutures are usually removed after 5–6 days and it is wise to check carefully that they are all out.

Care of Bladder and Bowel
The patient should pass urine on her own within 12 hours of delivery and the bladder should be properly emptied. If she does not pass urine in this time or appears to have partial retention she should be catheterized since retention predisposes to infection. Retention of urine occurs more frequently after complications and intervention at the time of delivery. When retention does occur it is wise to send a sample of urine for culture.

Constipation is common due to lack of exercise, reduced food and fluid intake in labour and perineal discomfort. Adequate fluid intake is important and if there is a problem the use of bran or bulk aperients such as normacol will usually solve it. Chemical aperients should be avoided as they cause colic and may be excreted in the milk, but suppositories are sometimes useful.

General Care

During the first part of the recovery period the mother should have adequate rest by night and day. In hospital many units have a rest period after lunch, when the mothers lie down for one and a half to two hours, it is wise to continue this practice at home. If the baby wakes the mother too much at night it may be sensible to move him into a separate room, though most mothers prefer to have their baby with them, and medically and pyschologically this is best. The mother should be up and about as soon as she has recovered from the delivery and certainly on the next day even if she has had a caesarean section. At home she should be relieved as far as possible of other responsibilities so that she can concentrate on her baby, particularly during the first two weeks. No special measures are required apart from the nursing observation.

Showers are better than baths and can be taken as soon after delivery as the woman wishes. There is no need for special vulval treatment but pads will be required for the lochia, and care should be taken to avoid the risk of genital tract infection by cleaning the perineum from front to back, and by avoiding introducing any unsterile object into the vagina.

At home and in many hospitals visiting is relatively unrestricted as friends and relatives naturally want to see the new baby. It is important to use common sense over this, since too many visitors can be tiring, and it is wise to restrict visiting so that mothers are not disturbed during their afternoon rest. Similarly anyone with an infection such as a cold or tonsillitis should keep away; this should be obvious but people are not always as considerate as one might expect.

It is during this time and particularly once she is at home that the mother gets to know her baby, learns the practical problems of looking after him and also first realizes how much hard work is involved if she has not had one before. The process of 'bonding' starts at delivery when she should hold her baby as early as possible and thereafter have as much contact as possible. The father should not be left out of this, but should be encouraged to hold the baby and join in the care and attention given to him. Similarly, other children should meet their new sibling as soon as they can and should be able to touch and, if they are old enough, to hold him.

Feeding

The mother should have decided whether she will feed the baby from breast or bottle before delivery. If she is going to breast-feed, the baby may be put to the breast briefly as soon as she wishes after delivery.* Initially the baby will receive only colostrum, the milk 'coming in' properly after approximately 48 hours when the breast may become tense and painful. (For details of feeding see Chapters 3 and 4.) The breasts must be well supported by a good brassière and the nipples treated carefully when washing; normal soap and water are adequate, but a little lanolin helps to keep the nipple soft and the skin intact.

If the mother does not wish to breast-feed or wishes to stop, the baby should not be put to the nipple and she must be warned against expressing milk as these manouvres stimulate lactation. A firm breast binder makes the breast more comfortable. There does not appear to be any advantage in increasing or restricting fluid intake. Oestrogens are generally avoided because of the risk of thromboembolism but bromocriptine, which acts by suppressing prolactin release (2.5 mg twice daily for two weeks), is an effective suppressant if one is needed.

Examination before leaving hospital or on the 9th or 10th day

This should include an overall assessment of the mother's well-being and particular note of the blood pressure, breast, abdomen and fundal height, perineum and vagina. It is wise to have the haemoglobin level checked before this examination. Since ovulation may occur within 6 weeks of delivery it is not too early to discuss contraception (see Chapter 15).

*For Lactation and Maternal Behaviour see Findlay, *Reproduction and the Fetus* Chapter 9.

Postnatal examination

This is usually done at 6 weeks and includes a check of blood pressure, breasts, abdomen, vagina and perineum. At this time a long-term contraceptive should be selected if this has not already been done.

During the puerperium the mother should do exercises to build up her stretched abdominal and perineal muscles. Advice on these is given in the antenatal classes and after delivery by physiotherapists or, more usually, midwives. They are of importance in helping the mother to be physically fit, and in restoring her figure and perineal muscles. Throughout the puerperium the mother needs support and advice.

After the initial joy of having her baby there sometimes follows a period of depression which normally resolves quickly; anxieties about the baby and relationships are very common. At this time and subsequently the mother needs help and understanding from family, friends and professionals with expert advice from the latter. The midwife, health visitor and general practitioner serve those at home; while midwives, obstetricians and paediatricians remain available for consultation.

Prevention of rhesus disease

Any rhesus negative woman without antibodies who gives birth to a rhesus positive infant is liable to be sensitized if fetal blood enters the maternal circulation. Cord blood is used to obtain the blood group of the neonate and if it is rhesus positive maternal blood is examined for the presence of fetal erythrocytes using the Kleihauer test. One-hundred μg Anti-D immunoglobulin given intramuscularly within 48 hour of delivery will normally prevent sensitization but, if the Kleihauer count is high, a larger dose may be advisable.

Notification of registration of birth (UK)

The midwife must notify the birth of any baby within 36 hours. The mother or father must register the baby with the Registrar of Births at the office for the area in which the baby was born within 6 weeks of birth.

Further reading

Mandel, P.E. (1981). *Breast-Feeding and Health*. Unicef, Geneva.

7

Complications in the puerperium

Serious complications in the puerperium are fortunately rare. There are many problems related to the baby which may worry the mother at this time but her own problems, if any, are usually minor. Nonetheless, expert advice is often needed and much of this is provided by midwives and health visitors; they or the patient may seek the doctor's advice, and it is important to take even minor problems seriously because of the strain on a new mother and in particular the risk of postnatal depression.

Puerperal pyrexia

This is defined as a pyrexia of 38°C occurring on two days within 14 days of delivery or miscarriage. It implies that there is an infection which must be diagnosed and treated, but investigation should begin as soon as the pyrexia is observed or there is any suggestion that the patient is unwell.

In the past puerperal fever, usually due to genital tract infection with *β haemolytic streptococci*, was common and caused the deaths of many women. With better obstetric care and understanding of the need to prevent infection the risk is greatly reduced and antibiotics are available to treat it when it occurs.

Infection may occur as follows:

1 Genital tract; Predisposing factors include long labour, obstetric interference and retained products of conception. Organisms which may be responsible include *E. coli,* bacteroides, staphylococci, anaerobic and haemolytic streptococcal organisms; occasionally clostridia may be involved.

2 Urinary tract; More likely to occur when the patient has had previous infection, catheterization during labour or retention of urine postpartum.

3 Breast; This is much less common than it was and is usually due to *Staphylococcus aureus.* It should be noted that a transient pyrexia often occurs after about 48 hours as lactation starts.

4 Respiratory tract; Usually occurs after anaesthesia or when the patient has an infection (not specific to pregnancy).

5 Deep vein thrombosis and thrombophlebitis

6 Other; It is important to remember that a pyrexia may be due to any of the causes which could occur apart from pregnancy or the puerperium.

Any patient with a pyrexia should be investigated as follows:

History
The obstetric or previous medical history, localized pain in the back (pyelonephritis), breast, leg or abdomen may suggest the likely cause of the pyrexia.

Examination
Should include inspection of the throat, infusion sites, breasts, abdomen, perineum and legs. In many cases the diagnosis is apparent. An offensive, heavy lochia suggests genital tract infection and in that event a swab should be taken.

Investigation
If there is no explanation for the pyrexia a high vaginal swab and midstream specimen of urine should be sent to the laboratory for culture and any other appropriate investigations undertaken.

Treatment
Will include appropriate antibiotics for infection and rest or mobilization as appropriate. In some cases of genital tract infection the uterus should be explored to remove, or exclude, the presence of retained products of conception. Abscesses, wherever they are should normally be drained, but some experience is required to decide when this is necessary with breast abscesses, and when it can be avoided. Prompt treatment with antibiotics usually avoids abscess formation. The painful breast should be supported and analgesics may be required. The baby should continue to feed from the other breast while the affected one should be emptied during the acute phase with a pump or by expression.

Other complications

Secondary postpartum haemorrhage (PPH)
This can occur any time after the first 24 hours and is defined as excessive blood loss from the genital tract. It usually occurs within 10 days of delivery and may take the form of a severe acute haemorrhage, though there is often an abnormal loss before this happens. The bleeding is due to retained products of conception, infection or both. If there is a pyrexia or suspicion of infection a high vaginal swab should be taken and antibiotics given before the uterus is explored to avoid the risk of septicaemia. Ergometrine, particularly if given intravenously may be helpful, but, if there is any doubt it is wise to

explore the uterus. If this happens to a patient at home it may be wise to call the local emergency obstetric team ('Flying squad').

Breakdown of the perineal repair

This may occur as a result of infection, haematoma or poor surgical technique. If possible the wound should be resutured, but this should be delayed if it is infected. The wound will often heal surprisingly well even if it is not resutured, but if it does not do so repair may be required later.

Haemorrhoids and anal fissures

These may cause problems which often start at the time of delivery when a fissure may occur or haemorrhoids prolapse. Thrombosis of a haemorrhoid may also occur at this time. Prevention by sparing the patient undue pushing in labour and avoiding constipation is important, and these conditions should be treated as they would be at any other time.

Dyspareunia (painful intercourse)

This is a later problem. A perineum which has been sutured will be tender for a few weeks but this should resolve by the time of the postnatal examination. If the repair is too tight or the scar remains painful at this stage, dilatation of the introitus, injection of local anaesthetic and hydrocortisone, or revision of the repair may be necessary according to the severity of the problem.

Psychological disorders

After delivery the mother is usually elated, but there is often considerable emotional lability during the first week. A period of depression (blues) often with crying, is common about the fifth day, when the understanding of family and staff is vital. A mother may feel inadequate and/or particularly anxious. Anxiety and depression are likley to be increased if there are difficulties with feeding the baby, or puerperal complications. Undiagnosed infections occasionally cause women to feel miserable. It is important to exclude an organic cause for malaise and not to attribute it to depression.

Any psychiatric disorder may present in relation to pregnancy or the puerperium, but the specific problem for which all involved with postnatal care must watch is puerperal depression. It is difficult to distinguish genuine mild postnatal depression from the postnatal blues, but more severe forms of depression are of a different order, and are potentially dangerous for mother and child. Most women who develop this disorder have no previous history of psychiatric disturbance and it may become apparent soon after delivery or, if it progresses slowly, weeks later when the health visitor may well identify it.

Symptoms and signs may include insomnia, nightmares, confusion, guilt about not loving the baby enough or 'being bad', loss of appetite, tearfulness, irritability and inability to cope with normal responsibilities. There is often undue anxiety over her own health and that of the baby and loss of sexual interest, hostility or indifference towards the husband. In severe cases the mother may harm herself or the baby. Expert psychiatric supervision is essential and there is a high risk, probably one in four, of recurrence in a subsequent pregnancy. Quite severe depression often goes unrecognized by all except the patient and it may lead to serious problems in the home, with marital disharmony and inadequate attention to the baby. Patients can sometimes describe vividly the gloom and desperation they felt while in this state and unable to get help.

Further reading

Anonymous (1979). *British Medical Journal,* **2**, 1487–88.

Sandler, M. Ed. (1978). *Mental Illness in Pregnancy and the Puerperium. Based on a symposium.* Oxford University Press, Oxford.

8

Statistics in relation to obstetrics

Statistics enable us to plan services and staffing, to assess the quality of care given to pregnant woman and babies, and to identify and remedy deficiencies. Comparison of international, national, area and unit statistics can help to identify differences in populations, risks and care, and to audit the performance of professionals at local level. But the reliability of information collected varies and it is important to remember how much populations, even within the same country or town can vary, as do staffing, facilities and standards. The provision of facilities and staffing, and the health of the population, depend on the standard of living and the racial characteristics of the inhabitants as well as on political decisions and administration. As yet there is no international agreement on definitions and this is essential if comparisons are to be valid.

The following are the most important, defined as in the UK

The birth rate
The number of births (live or stillbirths) after the 28th week of pregnancy per 1000 women aged 15–44.

Maternal mortality rate
The number of deaths occuring during pregnancy, during labour or as a consequence of pregnancy within one year of delivery or abortion per 100 000 births.

Direct deaths   are those due to obstetric complications, obstetric treatment or lack of it.

Indirect deaths   are those resulting from previous disease or disease developing during pregnancy and not due to an obstetric cause, but aggravated by pregnancy (previously described as 'associated deaths').

Fortuitous deaths   are those where disease occurred fortuitously in, or after pregnancy and was not related to the pregnancy (also previously 'associated deaths').

The WHO International Classification of Diseases includes only deaths up to 42 days after delivery or abortion.

Stillbirth rate
The number of babies stillborn (no sign of life and born after 28 weeks) per 1000 total births.

Neonatal mortality rate
The number of babies dying in the 28 days after birth per 1000 live births.

Perinatal mortality rate
The total number of stillbirths and deaths in the first seven days after delivery per 1000 total births.

Infant mortality rate
The number of infants dying in the first year of life per 1000 live births.

Much other information is available for example in relation to social class, legitimacy or illegitimacy and termination of pregnancy.

Maternal mortality

Confidential enquiries into maternal deaths in England and Wales started in 1952 and reports have been published for each three year period up to and including 1976–1978. The aim is to establish the cause of the death and whether it was 'avoidable' or not. This is done by collecting all the relevant details from the professional staff who were involved and passing the records to a regional obstetric,(and if appropriate anaesthetic) assessor before final assessment by statisticians and advisors at the Department of Health and Social Security. The confidentiality has enabled an increasingly high proportion (99 per cent in the last enquiry) of deaths to be investigated. There is concern that the number of deaths is now so low that cases may be identifiable from future reports, which might therefore be used in litigation.

Deaths may be due to a number of factors, but a main cause is selected on the evidence available and it is classified as a 'direct, indirect or fortuitous death'. Indirect deaths include those where pregnancy has exacerbated a non maternal disease or led to its diagnosis (See Table 8.1). (The maternal mortality rate at the beginning of the century was approximately 500 per 100 000 births.)

The deaths attributable to abortion were 14 in 1976–8; eight were due to legal abortion, 5 to illegal abortion and 2 to spontaneous abortion. Five other

Table 8.1 The main causes of maternal deaths directly due to pregnancy or delivery. From the maternal mortality report 1976–78.

Causes of death	Number or deaths
Pulmonary embolism	45 (25.7 per million maternities)
Hypertensive disease of pregnancy	29 (16.6 per million maternities)
Haemorrhage	26 (14.9 per million maternities)
Abortion	19 (10.9 per million maternities)
Other	227 (129.8 per million naternities)

direct obstetric deaths were due to anaesthetic complications during operations for abortion. Twenty-one were caused by ectopic pregnancy during the same period, and one woman with an ectopic pregnancy died from an anaesthetic complication.

The 1976–78 report is based on reports of 427 deaths, though in three of these cases no enquiry form was completed by the professional staff involved. The classification of these deaths was:

1. 227 (53 per cent) directly attributable to pregnancy or delivery.
2. 97 (23 per cent) indirectly attributable to pregnancy or delivery.
3. 103 (24 per cent) fortuitous.

The maternal mortality rate at the beginning of the century was approximately 5 per 1000 births and in 1976–78 it was 0.10 per 1000 total births (this rate excludes abortions). (Fig 8.1). The latest maternal mortality rates available for England and Wales, including death from abortion are 0.09 (1981) and 0.07 (1982).

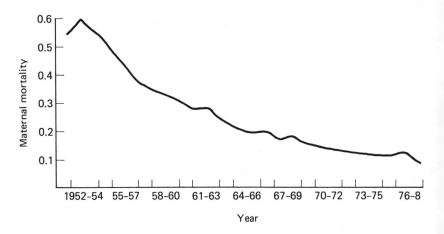

Fig. 8.1   Maternal mortality 1952–1978 (per 1000 maternities).

Perinatal mortality

The major causes of perinatal mortality are intrauterine hypoxia,RDS in low birthweight preterm infants, often complicated by an intraventricular haemorrhage (p.69), and congenital malformations. Malformations account for approximately 20 per cent of stillbirths and up to 40 per cent of neonatal deaths; 50 per cent of stillbirths show evidence of intrauterine hypoxia.

Figure 8.2 shows the fall which has occurred in perinatal and neonatal mortality from 1910–1982, and in proportion it has fallen faster in the last five years than in any previous five year period. The latest rate in England and Wales for 1982 for perinatal mortality is 11.3 per 1000 deliveries, with a stillbirth rate of 7.2 per 1000 deliveries and neonatal mortality (0–28 days) of 6.3 per 1000 live births. There is a wide range of perinatal and neonatal

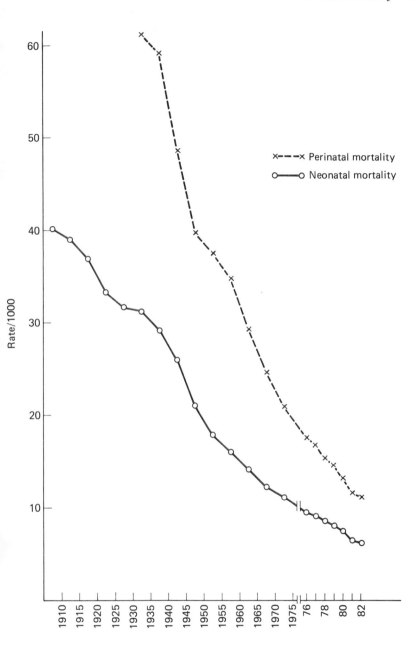

Fig. 8.2 Neonatal and perinatal mortality 1910–1982. Up to 1975 five-year averages are shown; thereafter single year data is presented.

mortality rates throughout the world, but caution is required in comparing rates in different countries or areas.

Not only are there differences between countries in the babies, particularly those weighing less than 1.00kg at birth, which actually get into the national statistics; but also the incidence of untreatable malformation such as anencephaly (Fig 8.3) varies enormously from country to country and may bias the perinatal data in a way that makes it difficult to evaluate the quality of perinatal care for viable infants. Furthermore, since the neonatal component of perinatal mortality is primarily a function of the incidence of low birthweight, and since this also varies widely both between and within countries (Table 8.2, and Fig. 8.4), it is one of the major determinants of intranational differences in the neonatal mortality rate.

For these reasons it has been suggested that perinatal mortality rate should be standardized for birthweight, and exclude infants with congenital malformations, since this would give a better indicator of the effectiveness of available health services.

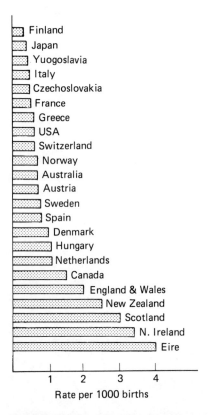

Fig. 8.3 Incidence of anencephaly in various countries (per 1000 total births). (With permission from Chalmers, I. and Macfarlane, A. (1980). Interpretation of Perinatal Statistics. In *Topics in Perinatal Medicine*. Edited by Wharton, B., Pitman Medical, London.)

Table 8.2 Incidence of low
birthweight (<2.50 kg) in
different countries.

India	28%
Malaysia	16.8%
Phillipines	14.2%
Cuba	10.8%
Hungary	10.8%
Singapore	7.4%
England	6.7%
USA	6.0%
Austria	5.7%
Japan	5.3%
Sweden	3.9%

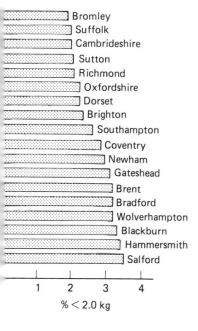

Fig. 8.4 Proportion of births weighing less than 2.0 kg in selected areas of England and
Wales. (With permission from Chalmers, I. and Macfarlane, A. (1980). Interpretation of
Perinatal Statistics. In *Topics of Perinatal Medicine*. Edited by Wharton, B. Pitman Medical,
London.)

A reduction in the number of low birthweight babies would make a major contribution to perinatal survival, and skilled neonatal care will improve the survival of those born with that low birthweight. The correlation of low birthweight with social class (Table 8.3) indicates how important improvement in economic, dietary and social factors could be in achieving this. Other factors contributing to low birthweight include preterm labour, medical induction of labour in the interests of maternal and fetal health, or intrauterine growth retardation. Smoking is another potentially avoidable factor associated with high perinatal mortality.

Table 8.3 The relationship of social class to birthweight and perinatal mortality

Social class	% with birthweight less than 2.50 kg (England and Wales 1980)	PNMR/1000 deliveries (England and Wales 1980)
I	5.3%	9.7
II	5.3%	11.1
III Non Manual	5.8%	12.8
III Manual	6.6%	12.8
IV	7.3%	15.0
V	8.1%	17.5

Obstetric disasters

Major disasters are fortunately uncommon and midwives and general practitioners can go through their careers without seeing anything go seriously wrong with one of their patients, though problems on the fetal side are more common. Reading the Maternal Mortality Reports is a good way of learning what can go wrong. Whenever there is a disaster, be it loss of a mother or baby, the effect on the parents, husband and the staff involved can be shattering. Emergencies can occur rapidly in obstetrics, and quick decisions and actions may be needed. However, many emergencies can be prevented and it is important to realize the danger of anaemia before labour, overstimulation of the uterus with syntocinon (particularly with multiparous patients) and inhalation of stomach contents during general anaesthesia; deaths from haemorrhage, amniotic embolus, ruptured uterus, Mendelson's syndrome and other caused are to be avoided.

If maternal death, stillbirth, neonatal death or severe congenital abnormality do occur, the first priority is to explain as far as possible what has happened, support the relatives and encourage others to do this. The birth of a child with severe abnormalities, whether it leads to death or not, may mean that there is a need for prolonged support, counselling about future pregnancy, and particularly close and sympathetic attention in any subsequent pregnancy and labour. There may also be decisions to be made about treatment for the neonate, a matter involving many individual, ethical and medical considerations. Finally when things go seriously wrong it is vital that the cause be established as far as possible in order to satisfy everyone involved and to minimize the risk of recurrence.

Further reading

Report (1982). *Report on Confidential Enquiries into Maternal Deaths in England and Wales 1976–78.* H.M.S.O. London.
Fofar, J.O. & Arneil, G.G.Ed. (1984). *Textbook of Paediatrics Vol.2* pp.1885-1894. Churchill Livingstone, Edinburgh.

Useful organizations

Stillbirth and Neonatal Death Society (SANDS)
Argyle House, 29-31 Euston Road, London NW1 2SD
Telephone: 01-833-2851/2
Foundations for the Study of Infant Deaths
3rd Floor, 4 Grosvenor Place, London SW1
Telephone: 01-235-1721

9

Abnormal pregnancy — early problems

Abortion

This is the expulsion of the products of conception from the uterus before the fetus is viable. Legally any fetus delivered dead after the 28th week in the UK is stillborn and must be registered as such, whereas before that it is aborted and registration is not required. With improved paediatric and obstetric care infants born before 28 weeks survive quite frequently and the limit could justifiably be 24 weeks. Any infant which breathes a breath counts as a live birth irrespective of its maturity. In the USA and Australia an abortion is defined as the end of a pregnancy before the 20th week. Abortions are generally described as occurring in about 15 per cent of pregnancies but measurements of chorionic gonadotrophin in early pregnancy suggest that the proportion may be as high as 50 per cent. The majority occur in the first trimester.

The causes of abortion

Most abortions occur because there is a blighted ovum (the gestation sac contains no embryo) or the fetus is abnormal. At least 30 per cent of aborted fetuses have chromosomal abnormalities. The commonest time is during the first trimester but abortions can occcur in the second trimester. Other causes of abortion include maternal infection and disease, multiple pregnancy, congenital abnormalities of the uterus, placenta praevia and cervical incompetence (see Table 9.1). In the latter case the cervix is weak and opens so that the membranes protrude into the vagina and rupture with subsequent expulsion of the fetus; characteristically this occurs in the second trimester, rapidly and with little pain. It is the result of damage to the internal cervical os by stretching, usually during the operation of dilatation of the cervix preparatory to curettage or termination of pregnancy.

The abortion can be prevented by putting a suture round the cervix to keep it closed; this was first described by Shirodkar and many people use this technique but there are others which are equally effective. The stitch is usually inserted at 14 weeks or thereabouts so that the chance of abortion due to other causes is reduced. It is removed a week or 10 days before the expected date of delivery unless there is reason to induce labour earlier or the uterus starts to

Table 9.1 The causes of spontaneous abortion and their timing.

	1st Trimester	2nd Trimester
Blighted Ovum	+	−
Fetal Abnormality	+	+
Uterine Abnormality	+	+
Chronic Disease e.g. renal, diabetes	+	+
Cervical Incompetence	−	+
Multiple Pregnancy	+	+
Placenta Praevia*	−	Occasionally
Acute Infection	Rarely	Rarely
Unexplained	+	+
Hydatidiform Mole	−	+
Ectopic Pregnancy	+ +	Rarely
Immunological Rejection (suspected)	+	+

*There is an increased likelihood of placenta prawvia if threatened abortion occurs.

contract strongly; strong contractions with the suture in place will eventually lead to tearing of the cervix or rupture of the uterus.

Diseases such as nephritis and diabetes are associated with a greater risk of abortion. Other factors which may lead to recurrent abortion (usually defined as three in succession) include uterine abnormalities (such as septum), chromosomal abnormalities of the parents, incompetent cervix and possibly immunological rejection. It is helpful to investigate the karyotype of the abortus and carry out a pathological examination when there is a history of repeated abortion.

Counselling after abortion

The loss of a baby even at an early stage is usually a cause of great distress and anxiety to the parents, particularly the mother. She needs to express her grief as she does if she loses a child. Discussion of the possible causes is helpful, both in relation to the loss of a pregnancy, for which the patient may blame the doctor or feel guilty herself and, in most cases, as reassurance for the future. Occasionally, as with recurrent abortion, investigations will be indicated. Generally there is no need to delay longer than couples wish before starting another pregnancy. It is sensible however, to advise couples to wait 3 months or as long as they feel is needed to get over the previous episode.

The odds are normally in favour of the next pregnancy being straightforward, but no one can predict the outcome of any conception; reassurance should be given but with a reservation to this effect. After conception sensible precautions include adequate rest, with the avoidance of fatigue, unusual or strenuous physical exertion, distant or stressful travel and sexual intercourse during the first trimester. Progestogens have been widely prescribed but there is no evidence that they are beneficial, though they may delay expulsion of a dead embryo or fetus. An early ultrasound examination will show if there is a live embryo, which is reassuring for patient and doctor, particularly if there has been a missed abortion before. Some of those who suffer abortions are pregnant unwillingly and their chief need afterwards is for good contraceptive advice.

Complete abortion

This means that all the products of conception have been expelled. The products should be kept for inspection if possible. After a complete abortion pain and bleeding cease, the cervix closes and the uterus contracts to become smaller and firmer. In this situation no treatment apart from reassurance and counselling for the future is required.

Incomplete abortion

Sometimes only some of the products of conception are expelled, for example the fetus alone. Examination of what has been expelled may indicate the diagnosis. Otherwise painful uterine contractions or bleeding may continue, or the retained tissue may become infected causing pain and pyrexia. On examination the cervix is open, sometimes with tissue in it while the uterus is large or bulky, according to the gestation and may also be tender. If an abortion is thought to be incomplete the uterus should be explored to remove any retained tissue; this should be done as soon as is conveniently possible to let the patient go home quickly, and to minimize the risk of haemorrhage and infection.

Threatened abortion

By definition, this occurs when a pregnant patient bleeds vaginally before 28 weeks. In the majority of those who have a threatened abortion the pregnancy

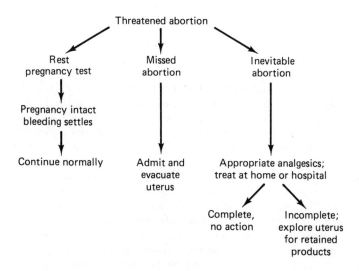

Fig. 9.1 The management of threatened abortion.

continues. The vaginal bleeding can vary from spotting to a heavy loss and there may be some ache or discomfort. Gentle pelvic examination will reveal that the uterus is appropriately enlarged and the cervix is closed. The treatment is rest, if possible in bed. In some cases the previous obstetric history, social circumstances or the amount of bleeding may justify admission to hospital. It is usual to advise rest in bed until 2 days after the bleeding stops and then the patient starts to get up and about again.

It is not unusual for dark (altered) blood to be lost for a few days after the fresh bleeding has stopped. (See Fig. 9.1). How long she should spend off work will depend on the severity of the episode, her home commitments, the nature of her work and the travelling involved, as well as the patient's own wishes in relation to the pregnancy.

Inevitable abortion

If the uterus is contracting strongly the likelihood is that abortion will occur. The cervix dilates and on examination products may be felt protruding through the cervix. Bleeding may be heavy. The pain and distress of an abortion is comparable to, and sometimes worse than that of a normal labour, so that appropriate analgesia and support will be required. Generally the abortion will progress steadily to a complete or incomplete abortion but, occasionally, it is justifiable in an early abortion to interfere surgically (for example when bleeding is severe).

Missed abortion

Occurs when the embryo or fetus dies but is retained with the other products of conception in the uterus. In this event there is often some loss of dark blood from the vagina and the uterus is small for the gestation period or does not increase in size between successive visits to the antenatal clinic. A negative pregnancy test is helpful but a false positive may be obtained and ultrasound examination may be more helpful. Uncertainty and delay are very distressing for the patient but observation over 5–7 days and repeat investigations may be required to confirm the diagnosis. The uterus will usually expel a missed abortion eventually, but the patient may find the wait intolerable, and there is a small risk of hypofibrinogenaemia. In most cases therefore, the obstetrician advises the patient to come into hospital for evacuation of the uterus or induction of abortion (usually with prostraglandins) according to the size of the uterus.

Complications of abortion

Haemorrhage
This may occur before, during or after the actual abortion. During the abortion it may be reduced if products distending the cervix are removed from it. Bleeding is a symptom and sign of incomplete abortion and the amount lost can be substantial; removal of retained tissue from the uterus is the remedy. Resuscitation and replacement of blood by transfusion of blood or other fluid

is carried out when required. Ergometrine (0.25–0.5 mg) given intravenously is a useful agent to produce uterine contraction. When severe bleeding occurs at home the 'flying squad' may be called to resuscitate and/or transfer the patient to hospital. In the rare cases when bleeding is heavy and the loss cannot be controlled by simple routine measures the possibility of an abnormal tendency to bleed should be considered. Where a dead fetus is retained in the uterus for four weeks or more hypofibrinogenaemia may occur. Rhesus negative women may be sensitized by fetal blood and should be given Anti-D (see p. 79).

Infection
This may occur in any abortion. In the past it was commonest after criminal abortion, relatively rare in the UK since the implementation of the Abortion Act in 1968. Now it is more likely when an abortion is incomplete, whether it occurred spontaneously or was induced. A variety of organisms may be responsible including *E. coli,* Streptococci and occasionally *Clostridium welchii* or *tetani*. On examination there is usually a pyrexia, the abdomen and uterus are tender and there may be an offensive purulent discharge from the cervix.

In severe infections which occur rarely, sometimes due to anaerobic organisms, there may be coma, jaundice or renal failure so that the patient needs close observation with investigation of the blood picture and measurement of the urinary output. Most infections are less severe and the principles of management include culture of swabs to identify the organisms responsible, evacuation of any retained products and the use of antibiotics in advance of surgical intervention so that the danger of Gram-negative septicaemia is prevented. Neglected infection may lead to damage to the tubes, subsequent infertility and chronic pelvic inflammatory disease.

Grief, depression and anxiety about future pregnancy
These are normal reactions to the loss of a pregnancy and the importance of giving explanation, reassurance and advice about the future has already been stressed. If the reaction is excessive or the loss of pregnancy occurs late, a psychiatrist may be helpful. Additional support may be needed during the next pregnancy, when the patient may be under considerable stress and in danger of confusing the second baby with the one she lost.

Injury to the genital tract
The vagina may be lacerated or perforated, the cervix torn or the uterus perforated. Haemorrhage and infection may follow these injuries, particularly after attempted criminal abortion. Occasionally the instrument used may perforate another viscus, such as bowel or bladder, or may be withdrawn with bowel or omentum attached. Chemical agents used for illegal abortion may cause infection or chemical peritonitis and salpingitis, while potassium permanganate causes severe vaginal ulceration and haemorrhage with subsequent scarring. Cervical incompetence as a result of undue dilatation of the cervix has already been described. In therapeutic termination of pregnancy (see Chapter 15) the danger relates directly to the duration of the pregnancy. (For the risk of death see Chapter 8, Maternal mortality).

Pathological examination

Material obtained when the uterus is evacuated should be examined histologically, with the fetus if it is recovered. Sometimes there is doubt about whether a woman was pregnant and the pathologist may help by confirming the presence of chorionic villi. Other abnormalities which relate to the pregnancy are occasionally found; these include trophoblastic disease, placental abnormalities and evidence of infection such as varicella, rubella, cytomegalovirus, listeriosis, malaria, syphilis and toxoplasmosis.

Ectopic pregnancy

This is the implantation of a pregnancy outside the normal uterine cavity. The commonest sites are:

1. The ampulla of the tube.
2. The isthmus of the tube.
3. The cornual angle of the uterus.

Others include the interstitial and fimbrial portions of the tube, the ovary, cervix and abdominal cavity (including the outside of the uterus). The latter are very rare and we should concentrate on tubal pregnancy. Ectopic pregnancies occur once in every 200–300 pregnancies. They are more likely in women who have had a previous ectopic (the chance of a second is about 10 per cent), in those who have an intrauterine device (about 1 in 30) and those who have had salpingitis or tubal surgery. They are thought to occur most frequently as a result of damage to the tube which produces adhesions, loss of cilia or fibrosis of the endothelium or muscle. In this way the lumen is blocked, or the lining or motility damaged so that implantation occurs where it should not.

The trophoblast invades the site of implantation and initially functions normally, producing chorionic gonadotrophin. The blood supply at the site of implantation is soon inadequate however, and the thin wall of the tube is liable to rupture (Fig. 9.2) so that these pregnancies rarely survive long.

Possible results are:

1. Tubal mole; there is haemorrhage round the embryo which dies and may subsequently be absorbed.

2. Tubal abortion; haemorrhage is followed by separation of part of the products and their passage along the tube.

3. Tubal rupture; the trophoblast erodes the tube until it ruptures and this may be accompanied, or followed, by severe haemorrhage.

4. Continuation of the pregnancy; this is very rare and can only occur when the implantation is on a site such as the external surface of the uterus where an adequate blood supply is available.

When the embryo dies there will normally be some bleeding vaginally as the decidua separates. Simultaneous ectopic and intrauterine pregnancies are seen occasionally.

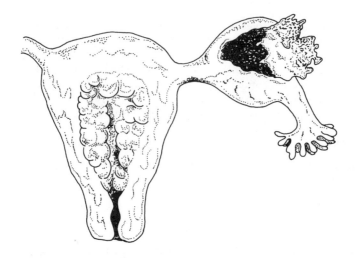

Fig. 9.2   Ruptured tubal preganncy with enlarged uterus showing decidua.

Presentation

An intact ectopic pregnancy may cause a little discomfort in the lower abdomen, usually on one side, and there is tenderness on the same side on pelvic examination. Bleeding into the tube or tubal abortion will be associated with more abdominal pain and tenderness, vaginal bleeding, and marked tenderness on one side of the pelvis and when the cervix is moved (cervical excitation pain). Sometimes a tender swelling can be detected but it is difficult to do this and too thorough an examination can rupture an ectopic pregnancy. Tubal rupture is dramatic and serious; the patient gets a sudden severe pain (sometimes like being kicked) and rapidly shows signs of shock and blood loss. If there is a lot of blood in the abdomen it may be distended, and a boggy mass of clotted blood felt behind the uterus.

Ectopic pregnancies can be difficult to diagnose. They must be differentiated from pelvic inflammatory disease (the diagnosis of unilateral pelvic inflammation is dangerous), threatened abortion, a bleed into or from a corpus luteum cyst, appendicitis and other causes of an acute abdomen. The patient often does not know she is pregnant, as the last period may have started only 4–6 weeks before, and there is usually little gastro-intestinal upset which helps to differentiate the condition from appendicitis. If there is cause to suspect an ectopic pregnancy it must be excluded, usually by laparoscopy or laparotomy. Ultrasound examination is helpful but not totally reliable, and ordinary pregnancy tests are often negative. Paracentesis may be helpful if laparoscopy is not possible since the presence of blood will make the diagnosis very likely. The usual treatment is salpingectomy (removal of the affected tube), though it is sometimes possible to preserve the tube and conservative operations are being used increasingly. If the patient has severe haemorrhage this must be stopped urgently; the surgeon cannot afford to wait until blood is available and resuscitation is only possible once the haemorrhage has been stopped. This is a dangerous condition, often misdiagnosed, which contributes to maternal mortality (see p. 86).

Hydatidiform mole

This is a rare condition in this country, though it is commoner in the Far East and West Africa. In almost all cases there is no fetus. The condition which occurs in Caucasians approximately once in every 2000 pregnancies is thought to be the result of two sperm fertilizing an oocyte, or of abnormal spermatozoa. The incidence rises in older women. Usually the mole has a female karyotype and consists of a mass of fluid filled cysts about the size of currants, but classically described as 'a bunch of grapes.' The tumour is functional; it produces chorionic gonadotrophin and invades endometrium in the same way as normal trophoblast (Fig. 9.3).

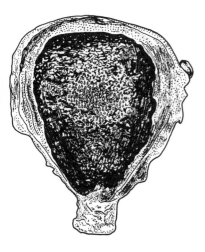

Fig. 9.3 Hydatidiform mole.

Presentation and diagnosis

Excessive vomiting is often the first symptom of a mole and subsequently women present with vaginal bleeding and abdominal pain, typically between the 12th and 16th week. Occasionally hypertension occurs and a patient may present with pre-eclampsia. The uterus is larger than normal for the duration of the pregnancy in at least half the patients; of the remainder half have an average sized, and half a small uterus. Tenderness of the uterus is common. In some cases vesicles are passed from the cervix, or abortion of the mole occurs. Otherwise the diagnosis may be suspected by the finding of abnormally high hCG levels and the absence of a fetal heart confirmed by ultrasonic examination (which gives a characteristic appearance like a snowstorm.

Management

The tumour is usually evacuated by suction as in termination of pregnancy; it is important to have blood cross-matched as bleeding can be profuse and it is particularly easy to perforate the uterus.

About 2 per cent of moles develop into chorioncarcinoma and careful supervision is mandatory for 2 years. During this time urine, serum or both are used for hCG measurements and pregnancy should be avoided as it confuses the situation. The hCG level should come down to normal level, if it does not do so there must be viable trophoblast, which may have undergone malignant change.

Chorioncarcinoma

This is a rare condition which can be highly malignant and occurs during pregnancy or after pregnancy or abortion. Half the cases follow hydatidiform mole so that it is similarly commoner in the Far East and the African continent. These cases should be diagnosed as a result of surveillance after abortion or evacuation of the mole. Some moles persist or are locally invasive and these are nowadays treated in the same way as chorioncarcinoma. The remainder follow, or coincide with pregnancies or abortion; they may be diagnosed as a result of persistent abnormal bleeding or may present with symptoms attributable to metastases in the lungs, brain, bowel, genital tract or elsewhere. The level of hCG will reveal the diagnosis.

The tumour is often highly invasive and metastasizes rapidly. Metastases and primary sites may bleed profusely and death can occur quickly. The modern treatment, which is remarkably successful considering the vicious nature of the tumour involves courses of chemotherapeutic agents such as methotrexate and actinomycin D. The response is monitored by changes in the levels of hCG, with radiological or other investigations where appropriate. At least 75 per cent of patients should be cured, the main problem being those who present with advanced disease. After cure reproductive function is normally preserved. In very rare cases their tumour can occur on the ovary (as it does in the testis and mediastinum).

Further reading

Miller, J.F., Williamson, E., Glue, J., Gordon, Y.B., Grudinskad, J.G. and Sykes, A. (1980). Fetal Loss After Implantation: a prospective study. *Lancet*, **ii**, 554–6.

Potter, E.L. and Craig, J.M., (1976). *Pathology of the Fetus and Infant.*

Short, R.V. (1979). When a Conception Fails to Become a Pregnancy, Ciba Foundation Symosium, Amsterdam, *Experta Medica*, 377–94.

Westrom, L, Bengtsson, L.P.H. and March, P.A. (1981). Incidence, Trends and Risks of Pregnancy in a Population of Women. *British Medical Journal*, **i**, 15–18.

10

Abnormal pregnancy — later problems

Antepartum haemorrhage (APH)

Bleeding from the genital tract during the period from the 28th week to delivery. The causes are:

Placenta praevia
A placenta attached partly or wholly to the lower uterine segment (maternal bleeding).

Abruptio placentae
Separation of a placenta normally situated in the upper uterine segment (maternal bleeding).

Vasa praevia
(Rare) from a vessel running in, or attached to the membranes over the internal os where there is a velamentous insertion (fetal bleeding).

Other
From local conditions such as carcinoma of the cervix, cervical polyp, erosion, vaginitis and vulval varices.

Placenta praevia

This is graded according to the extent to which the placenta encroaches on the lower segment (see Fig. 10.1). It is commoner with multiple pregnancy (because the placenta is larger) and after caesarean section. Bleeding can occur at any time and in a few patients occurs before 28 weeks (when it is classified as threatened abortion). It may follow coitus, examination or external version (see p. 112). The placenta tends to be sheared off as the lower segment forms, typically causing fresh, painless bleeding which is likely to recur. The lie may be oblique or transverse and the presenting part high when there is a significant portion of the placenta in the lower segment, while an anterior placenta may make palpation of the presenting part difficult. Bleeding does not always occur before labour, particularly with Type IV. The diagnosis is now often made by ultrasound before haemorrhage has occurred.

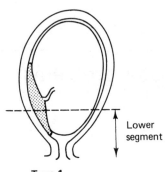

Lower
segment

Type 1
Does not reach
the internal os.

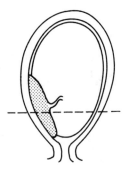

Type 2
Margin reaches the internal os.

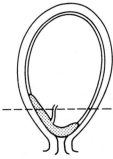

Type 3
Overlies the internal os.

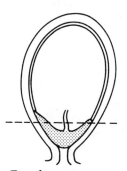

Type 4
Overlies the internal os
and would do so if it
were fully dilated.

Fig. 10.1   Classification of placenta praevia.

If a patient suffers an antepartum haemorrhage she should be admitted to hospital (if appropriate by the emergency obstetric team), and placenta praevia is the presumptive diagnosis if it is not abruption of the placenta (see p. 103). In hospital the woman's general and obstetric condition should be assessed. If she is well and the bleeding not heavy, she is treated by bed rest and observation. Vaginal examination is contraindicated because it may cause or increase bleeding, but many obstetricians favour a speculum examination to see if there is any lesion of the cervix or lower genital tract when the bleeding is not heavy. It is wise to check the haemoglobin and cross match 2 units of blood which should be kept, or replaced, until delivery. The diagnosis should be established within 24–48 hours preferably by ultrasound. If this is not available isotope scanning or radiography may be used. If placenta praevia cannot be excluded in any other way the patient should be examined under anaesthesia in theatre at 38 weeks. There should be a drip running, blood available and staff ready to proceed to immediate caesarean section as examination may cause heavy bleeding. If the placenta is praevia it is usual to proceed to caesarean section. If the placenta is not felt the membranes may be ruptured to allow labour to proceed.

When a major degree of placenta praevia (Type III or IV) is established, caesarean section is obligatory. In doubtful cases examination under anaesthesia may still be justified and in minor cases of anterior placenta praevia, particularly if labour has started, it may be justifiable to allow labour to proceed. If bleeding is severe or there is fetal distress, early caesarean section is indicated.

Most patients with placenta praevia stop bleeding after the first episode. They must, however, stay in hospital until they are delivered. Placenta praevia is the diagnosis with antepartum haemorrhage unless or until it is excluded. Anyone with known or suspected placenta praevia must be kept in hospital. This is not welcome advice for healthy pregnant women, who may have young children at home, and it is vital to explain precisely why it is unsafe for them to leave hospital.

Abruptio placentae

The bleeding may be revealed or concealed. In the latter case it is collected behind part of the placenta and there is pain, which may be severe and associated with shock. Bleeding from the margin of the placenta may be painless and indistinguishable from that due to placenta praevia. If there is concealed bleeding there will be tenderness over the affected part of the uterus, which may be mild or severe according to the degree of abruption. With greater severity the uterus is firm or tense, and if there has been a large haemorrhage the fundus may be higher than previously, while palpation of the fetus and auscultation of the fetal heart may be impossible.

Labour often starts and the fetus may be distressed or dead as a result of the placental damage. In most cases there is no explanation for abruption but it is more likely to occur with hypertension or trauma and occasionally follows the sudden loss of a large amount of liquor.

If she is at home the patient should be admitted to hospital, and the 'flying squad' called if there is a long journey or the abruption is severe. An intravenous infusion should be started, blood cross-matched and the haemoglobin checked. Disseminated intravascular coagulation may occur, with consumption of coagulation factors and fibrinogen, and the danger of abnormal bleeding. Expert haematological advice may be required but observation of the readiness with which a blood sample clots in a glass tube may give a useful indication of whether this is a problem.

If there is a clotting disorder it must be corrected. If the fetus is alive many obstetricians favour caesarean section as speedily as possible, though some advocate rupturing the membranes and allowing labour to proceed, which is certainly the best course if the fetus is dead. If the fetus is alive its condition should be monitored closely. There is a particular risk of postpartum haemorrhage as a result of coagulation disorder; therefore the general condition, blood pressure, pulse, urine output and oxygenation of the patient should be observed carefully. There is a serious risk to the mother from haemorrhage, and to the fetus from prematurity and hypoxia.

Polyhydramnios

This is an excess of amniotic fluid. Normally the amount increases until approximately 36 weeks, reaching a maximum of about 800 ml*. An excess may be detected at any time from 24 weeks, but the amount must be considerably in excess of the normal before it is detectable clinically. The volume can be calculated from ultrasound measurement. The distension of the abdomen, the abdominal girth, the tone and size of the uterus and difficulty in palpating fetal parts help detection.

In over half the cases no abnormality is found to explain the hydramnios. It may be due to fetal abnormality, notably open neural tube defects, exomphalos, upper gastrointestinal atresia, or hydrops fetalis. Multiple pregnancies, particularly uniovular twins, are associated with excess liquor and rarely it is due to the presence of a placental tumour. The most important maternal cause is diabetes, though it occurs with cardiac, hepatic or renal disease.

The liquor usually accumulates slowly but it may do so acutely, particularly in the second trimester with uniovular twin pregnancy when there may be quite severe abdominal pain and vomiting and there is a serious risk of premature labour. Possible causes of an excess of liquor should be excluded by ultrasound, X-ray and glucose tolerance test as appropriate.

Unstable or abnormal lie, abnormal presentation and premature labour are all more common when there is hydramnios. The risk of cord prolapse is greater, as are placental abruption, amniotic embolus and postpartum haemorrhage. In acute hydramnios or if the patient is very uncomfortable because of the quantity of fluid it may be justifiable to reduce the volume by abdominal paracentesis, though it may recur.

Oligohydramnios

The liquor decreases when the placenta is functioning inadequately for the fetus as seen most frequently with postmaturity. Rarely the fetus has renal agenesis or an obstruction to the output of urine and the fetus shows abnormalities attributable to the pressure of the uterus. Before term, any suggestion that there is scanty liquor should prompt investigation of fetal well-being and normality.

Abdominal pain in pregnancy

Many women suffer mild or disturbing abdominal pain during pregnancy and it is important to distinguish this from pain indicating disease or complications of pregnancy. Pain may occur as a result of uterine contraction, bowel distension (common in the first trimester), the position of the fetus (e.g. head

*See Findlay, Reproduction and the Fetus, Fig. 7.8, p. 113.

under the costal margin) or in the groins, when it is attributed to stretching of the round ligaments, though it is difficult to justify this explanation. The most important obstetric causes of serious pain are ectopic pregnancy and abruption of the placenta, though it may be due to degeneration of a fibroid, rupture of the uterus or acute hydramnios. Other causes include hiatus hernia, appendicitis, haemorrhage into, or torsion of an ovarian cyst and all the other causes of acute abdominal pain which may occur in pregnancy as well as out of it.

Acute appendicitis illustrates the problems of diagnosis in pregnancy since its position changes as the uterus enlarges; it may be much higher in the abdomen than normally and situated behind the uterus. The signs and symptoms are different and may be confusing, particularly when the tenderness is found high or laterally in the abdomen instead of in the region of McBurney's point. If the appendix is behind or adherent to the uterus this organ may be tender, suggesting a different diagnosis.

Pre-eclampsia

This is a disorder of pregnancy traditionally diagnosed by the presence of any two of these characteristic features: oedema, hypertension and proteinuria. This definition is no longer acceptable as oedema occurs frequently among pregnant women and although it may be severe in pre-eclampsia, it is not present in every case. In many cases there is only hypertension but some women develop proteinuria and of these a few may progess to eclampsia (see p. 107). It is important to know the blood pressure of a woman when not pregnant or in early pregnancy to distinguish pre-eclampsia from other causes of hypertension. A rise of the diastolic to 90 mmHg in a previously normotensive patient indicates the need for investigation and treatment.

The disease is common in primigravid women and those with obesity, diabetes, hypertension, multiple pregnancy or hydatidiform mole. There is a familial tendency, and there are racial and geographical variations.

Many theories have been proposed to explain pre-eclampsia including dietary factors, excessive salt intake, a pressor effect of various hormones produced in the placenta, an immunological response, disseminated intravascular coagulation (which is probably secondary rather than primary), loss of normal insensitivity to increased levels of angiotension II found in pregnant women, and a disturbance of the ratio of vasodilatory and vasoconstricting prostaglandins and prostacyclins.

The disease may be mild, moderate or severe, and may progress rapidly or slowly or remain static for a long period. Hypertension, particularly if it progresses to eclampsia, increases the risk to the mother and to the fetus. There is reduced maternal blood flow through the choriodecidual space and there are increased rates of perinatal death, growth retardation and premature delivery.

Management

This depends on the degree of the disease and the wellbeing of the fetus. Close observation of the mother and fetus is essential to establish their condition and to identify any change. In moderate to severe cases this is likely to involve hospital admission. Some women with mild disease may be able to stay at home provided they can rest, and there is adequate regular observation arranged by midwife, general practitioner and hospital, and no sign of complications or progression. In other patients, paticularly those who have been overactive, blood pressure settles and may even return to normal after a short rest in hospital enabling them to return home, though the pre-eclampsia may recur. A relatively small rise in blood pressure may be very significant in pregnancy, when it would not be in relation to the normal medical mangement of hypertension. Proteinuria is generally a sign of serious and increasing disease.

The woman is not confined to bed unless she has severe pre-eclampsia. The degree of rest must be related to the severity of the disease which often shows improvement with the initial hospital rest. In severe disease when there is a danger of eclampsia the patient should be treated with intensive care by a team of nurses, obstetricians and anaesthetists in an area where there is an absence of noise, bright lights and other disturbance since external stimuli can provoke eclamptic fits.

Drugs

In mild disease these are not necessary. Diuretics are not now regarded as helpful in most cases and sedatives are not given as they depress the mother and fetus. Hypotensive drugs are being used increasingly and methyldopa is the usual choice though labetalol and other α and β blocking preparations are being used. In severe disease when eclampsia threatens and control of the blood pressure is required urgently, intravenous hydralazine (40 mg in 500 ml 5 per cent dextrose) is suitable but diazoxide, reserpine and other preparations can be used. (The prevention of convulsions is described under eclampsia.)

Observations

Blood pressure taken daily in mild cases, 4-hourly or more frequently otherwise. Fluid intake and urinary output except in mild cases.

Investigations

1. Microscopy and culture of the urine (to exclude other cases of proteinuria).
2. Urinary protein (quantified).
3. Blood urea (raised levels indicate impaired renal function).
4. Serum creatinine (raised levels indicate impaired renal function).
5. Serum uric acid (rises with moderate or severe disease).
6. Assessment of fetal growth and wellbeing by ultrasound, fetal movement chart, cardiotocography, biochemical methods (see p. 9).

Induction of labour or caesarean section

The danger from pre-eclampsia to mother or fetus, the problems of induction and delivery and the dangers of prematurity have to be balanced in deciding when intervention is justified. When there is a real danger of eclampsia intervention is almost always justified. The blood pressure may go up during labour or after delivery, and it is wise either to reduce the dose of ergometrine to 0.25 mg at the end of the second stage or to rely on oxytocin alone.

Eclampsia

This term is used when convulsive fits occur in a patient with pre-eclampsia (see also p. 105). In the past eclampsia was a major cause of maternal death, but now only 1 in 50 dies, and the risk of perinatal fetal death is approximately 5 per cent. Maternal complications include cerebral haemorrhage, anoxia, renal failure, hepatic failure, and disseminated intravascular coagulation. The fits are ascribed to the severe cerebral oedema usually found, and cerebral hypoxia.

Symptoms and signs

Those which may occur when eclampsia is imminent include severe headache, visual disturbance, epigastric pain, vomiting, restlessness, irritability and drowsiness. Severe oliguria, and a rapid increase in blood pressure or oedema are also significant. Anuria is particularly sinister.

Prevention

It should be possible to prevent fits occuring by reducing the stimuli which trigger them, lowering the blood pressure and giving an anticonvulsant. It is desirable to deliver the baby as soon as the disease is controlled.

The anticonvulsant should, preferably, be one which does not have adverse effects on the fetus. Magnesium sulphate is effective and has been used for many years; 10–12 ml of a 50 per cent solution (5–10 g) intramuscularly initially and then 5–10 ml every 4–6 hours is one regime, or an intravenous injection of 5–10 g can be given followed by a continuous infusion of 2–4 g every hour. It is important to maintain the urinary output and to ensure that the patient is not over depressed by checking the respiration rate (which should exceed 12/min) and the intensity of the knee jerks. If available, measurement of serum levels is an advantage, 6–8 mmol/litre is optimal. Chlormethiazole (an anticonvulsant and sedative) is given intravenously using a 0.8 per cent solution, 50–100 drops per minute to obtain control which is maintained by 20–30 drops per minute. Oversedation leads to unconsciousness and respiratory depression. The solution is unstable at tropical temperatures. Intravenous diazepam 10–20mg followed by further doses if necessary gives good control but depresses the fetus and has a half life of over 90 hours. Other drugs used include thiopentone, omnopon, morphine, paraldehyde and combinations of drugs such as pethidine, promazine and chlorpromazine. The choice depends upon the staff available, the gravity of the situation, the health of the fetus and the experience of the team concerned with particular drugs. Magnesium sulphate has stood the test of time and remains popular, particularly in the United States of America.

Emergency Treatment of Eclampsia

If fits do occur, there is a tonic stage with general spasm and cyanosis, a clonic stage of alternate spasm and relaxation followed by a period of coma. Fits may occur at any interval and during the clonic stage there is considerable risk of injury. Morphine is useful as an emergency measure or for transportation. It is often helpful to give a rapidly acting diuretic such as frusemide intravenously to reduce oedema. Emergency treatment includes; the insertion of a gag or airway (on which the patient can bite), suction of the airway and administration of oxygen. As soon as possible the situation should be controlled with anticonvulsant (see treatment of pre-eclampsia) and hydralazine given intravenously. The patient is then nursed in the labour ward or an intensive care unit with the minimum of noise and disturbance. Catheterization is important to avoid the stimulus of a full bladder and to measure the urinary output. An epidural or caudal anaesthetic is ideal if the patient is in labour.

Other nursing care includes normal measures for an unconscious patient and quarter-hourly observations, or continuous monitoring of patient and fetus. If the patient is to be moved any distance she should be accompanied by a doctor and, preferably, a full emergency squad.

If vaginal delivery occurs the second stage should be shortened with the forceps or ventouse. The paediatricians should be informed of the patients's condition so that they can be prepared for the delivery and be present. It is wise to check for disseminated intravascular coagulation.

After delivery the measures are continued for 48 hours or until the disease improves, as judged by the general condition, blood pressure, oedema and urinary output. The blood pressure may take days or weeks to revert to normal, or may not do so at all; almost all these patients have hypertension later in life.

Multiple pregnancy

The incidence of twins is approximately 1 in 80, triplets 1 in 80^2 and quadruplets 1 in 80^3. However, the chances are increased for negroes (they are decreased for Asians) and for those treated with drugs to stimulate ovulation (clomiphene and gonadotrophins but not bromocriptine). Twins may be monovular (or monozygotic), when the babies will be identical, or binovular. For each binovular twin there will be a separate placenta, amnion and chorion; but monovular twins may share chorion, amnion and placenta. In the latter case the circulations may connect and one fetus may thrive at the expense of the other. There is a familial tendency to have binovular twins, the risk increasing in older women.

Symptoms and complications of twin pregnancy

These are increased for triplets and quadruplets. They include:

In the first trimester;   increased vomiting, large uterus for dates, increased risk of abortion.

In the second trimester;   vomiting may continue, uterus large for dates, polyhydramnios, abortion, presence of multiple fetal parts, anaemia.

Third trimester;   uterus large for dates, polyhydramnios, malpresentation, abnormal lie, anaemia, antepartum haemorrhage, pre-eclampsia, premature labour, pressure symptoms (gastrointestinal, varicose veins, oedema, dyspnoea).

Labour; premature, fetal malpresentation, cord prolapse, slow progress, retained placenta, postpartum haemorrhage.

Puerperium; twice the work for mother feeding and caring for two babies.

In addition there is a increased risk of fetal abnormality (particularly with monovular twins), intrauterine asphyxia, growth retardation and complications. Therefore the risk of virtually every complication of pregnancy and labour is increased.

The diagnosis nowadays is often made by ultrasound early in pregnancy (Fig. 10.2). Otherwise it may be suspected because of the features mentioned above, most commonly because the uterus is large for dates. Confirmation by ultrasound or X-ray is required; this determines the number of fetuses and excludes some possible abnormalities.

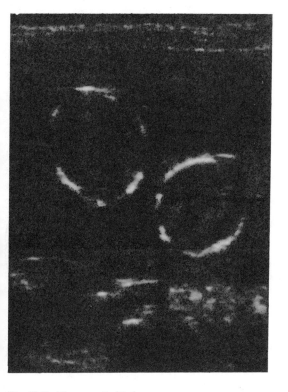

Fig. 10.2 Ultrasound of twin pregnancy.

Early diagnosis enables the patient to be advised of the need for rest and particular care, and to be given iron and folic acid. Booking should be at a hospital with full facilities because of the risk of complications. Admission from 28–32 weeks is practised at some hospitals to reduce the risk of prematurity but there is no evidence this is effective. It is important to admit any woman who develops complications. By 38 weeks most are delivered. If not delivered they may be showing growth retardation, or the mothers are so uncomfortable they welcome admission to hospital and induction at the appropriate time, and not later than term.

The common lies and presentation are shown in Figure 10.3. One fetus splints the other so spontaneous version (the baby turning to a different presentation on its own) is rare and external version by an obstetrician is contraindicated.

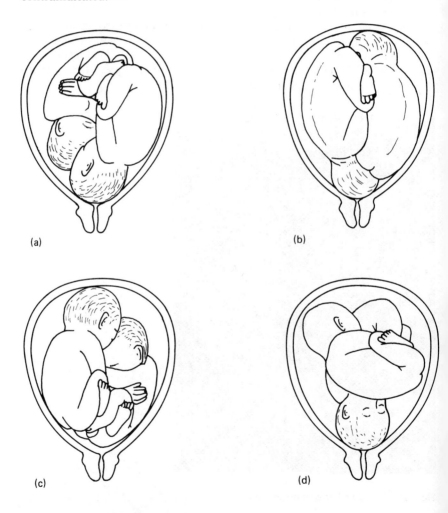

(a)   (b)

(c)   (d)

Fig. 10.3 Presentation of twins: (a) both cephalic; (b) one cephalic, one breech; (c) both breech and (d) one transverse, one cephalic.

Labour

This may be longer than average, and both fetuses should be monitored throughout. Difficulty at delivery is most likely to arise with the second twin and therefore an experienced obstetrician, anaesthetist and paediatrician should be present. An epidural block is helpful if the delivery is difficult and avoids the risk of giving a general anaesthetic in unfavourable situations between deliveries. The first twin is delivered in the normal way. Immediately afterwards the lie, presentation and fetal heart rate of the remaining twin must be checked. If the lie is abnormal it can usually be corrected. When a contraction occurs and the presenting part descends, the membranes should be ruptured and the baby delivered. There is a risk of fetal hypoxia as the uterus contracts and of cord prolapse if the presentation is abnormal. Forceps are used if appropriate. Where there is fetal distress, an abnormal lie or other indication for caesarean section before or during labour this should be done; it may be particularly appropriate if the twins are very premature.

Rarely twins are not diagnosed until after delivery of the first. If the oxytocic has been given the risk to the retained twin is considerable and the lie should be checked, corrected if necessary, the membranes ruptured and delivery expedited. Postpartum haemorrhage is more likely after twin delivery, and, if the uterus is hypotonic, a continuous oxytocin infusion will prevent this.

Abnormal lie

The lie may be oblique, transverse or unstable, and all are commoner in multigravid rather than in primigravid women. The lie may be abnormal because of a congenital abnormality of the uterus, a fibroid or ovarian cyst in the pelvis, polyhydramnios, placenta praevia, fetal abnormality or uterine laxity.

The lie is determined by palpation and there may be a known or recognizable aetiology, though it may be necessary to exclude placenta praevia and fetal abnormality by ultrasound or X-ray. If there is no contraindication an attempt may be made to correct the lie by external version. If the lie is not corrected after 36 weeks, it is wise to admit the patient to hospital until the lie is corrected or until she has had her baby. If the membranes rupture or she goes into labour with an unstable lie the cord may prolapse and obstructed labour will occur. Unless the lie can be corrected delivery by caesarean section is unavoidable. When this abnormal lie is due to laxity of the uterus, it may correct spontaneously when the fetus is larger, the liquor less and uterine tone increased.

Breech presentation

This means the buttocks lie in, or immediately above the pelvis instead of the head. At 28 weeks approximately 25 per cent of fetuses present by the breech but the majority will correct spontaneously to a cephalic position, leaving about 3 per cent as term approaches. A fetus presenting by the breech may not be able to undergo spontaneous version because of:

1. Congenital abnormality of the uterus (septate or bicornuate).
2. Multiple pregnancy; where one twin 'splints' the other.
3. Fetal abnormality particularly hydrocephalus.
4. Lack of liquor.
5. Extension of its legs.
6. An 'obstruction' such as a fibroid or ovarian cyst.

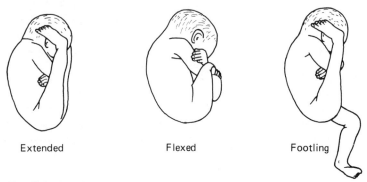

Extended   Flexed   Footling

Fig. 10.4   Breech presentation.

The breech presentations are described as extended, flexed or footling (see Fig. 10.4). Extended breeches occur most frequently in primigravida. The position is described in relation to the sacrum (left or right, anterior or posterior). The management of breech presentation is controversial at the present time.

External Version

It is often possible for the obstetrician to correct the presentation to cephalic by external version and such a policy does reduce the incidence of breech delivery. Version is often easy at 32 weeks or soon after, but if it is left too late it will be impossible; the optimum time is 32–36 weeks. As many obstetricians now advise caesarean section for breech presentation there is a logical argument for trying to prevent this.

External version is contraindicated by multiple pregnancy, hypertension, antepartum haemorrhage, large fibroids, known congenital abnormalities of the uterus, some abnormalities (e.g. hydrocephalus), or fetal death, and in those cases destined to have a caesarean section in any case. Version can be associated with placental separation, rupture of the membrane, cord entanglement, and feto–maternal bleeding. Complications should not occur if the version is attempted, as it should be, only gently, in unanaesthetized patients without any of the contraindications mentioned above. The fetal heart should be checked before and after version and the vulva inspected for bleeding or loss of liquor.

Risks of Breech Delivery

Delivery of a fetus is more hazardous with a breech than it is with a cephalic presentation because if any cephalo-pelvic disproportion becomes apparent it is too late for caesarean section. There is also an increased risk of asphyxia, due to cord compression and reduced placental blood flow at the time of delivery. Additionally there is little time for moulding of the head. Cord prolapse may occur during labour, particularly with a flexed breech. Causative abnormalities and the higher proportion of breech presentation in premature labours add to the morbidity and mortality associated with breech delivery.

Diagnosis and Route of Delivery

The diagnosis of a breech is not always as easy as might be expected, and if in doubt leaving the hand gently on the fundus for a minute or two will often help because fetal movement demonstrates that the breech is at the fundus. Vaginal examination usually leaves no doubt about the presenting part.

The route of breech delivery is also controversial and there is an increasing tendency towards caesarean section particularly for primigravidae. Caesarean section is indicated, provided the fetus is normal, if there is a uterine scar, or any doubt about the adequacy of the pelvis; any other factors such as prematurity, maternal age or long infertility must be considered in deciding the method of delivery. If there is any question of vaginal delivery the fetus and pelvis must be carefully assessed by an experienced obstetrician, as well as by X-ray pelvimetry and ultrasound. It should be remembered that there are dangers from caesarean section for mother and baby.

Mechanisms of Delivery

The position of the breech leads to engagement of the bitrochanteric diameter (9–10 cms) in the transverse axis. Subsequently the pelvis will rotate anteriorly, and lateral flexion enables the pelvis of the fetus to pass through the birth canal. The breech is then delivered in the lateral position and restitution to the sacro-anterior position follows. With delivery of the trunk the shoulders engage in the transverse diameter and external rotation occurs as a result. The shoulders will follow the same mechanism as the breech and trunk, rotating to the antero-posterior axis before delivery, and with continuing descent the head will also engage in the transverse diameter and rotate internally. The head may be deflexed due to the resistance of the tissues of, and surrounding, the birth canal. If there is a lack of progress or failure of the breech to engage caesarean section is advisable.

Some degree of assistance is required in breech delivery to minimize the risks. There is a tendency for the patient to bear down before the cervix is fully dilated, this must be prevented by encouragement to resist the urge, epidural anaesthesia, or rasing the foot of the bed. Vaginal examination to exclude cord prolapse after rupture of the membranes is essential and there should be close monitoring in case this happens subsequently. It is vital that the procedure for the breech delivery be explained carefully in advance to the patient as it is quite different from normal delivery.

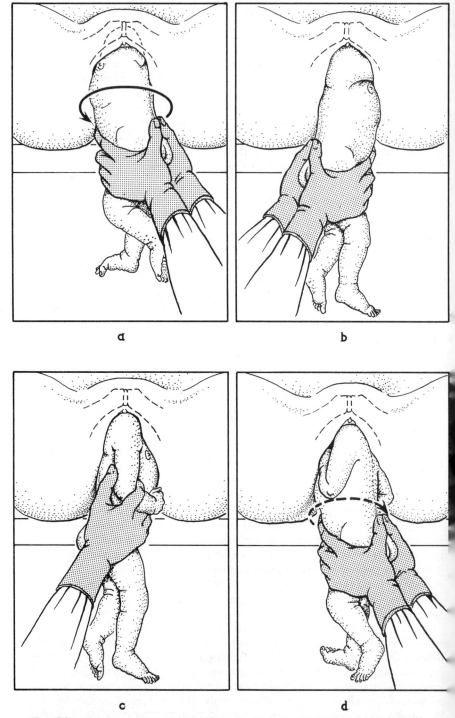

Fig. 10.5 Løvset's manoeuvre: (a) the baby is rotated through 180°; (b) the posterior (right) shoulder is anterior and below the pubis; (c) the shoulder is delivered, then (d) the trunk is rotated the other way through 180° to bring the other (left) shoulder below the pubis. (With kind permission from Sir Stanley Clayton, reproduced from *Obstetrics by Ten Teachers* 13th edn. (1980). Edward Arnold, London.)

The principles of vaginal breech delivery

1. With an obstetrician, anaesthetist and paediatrician present, the patient is placed in the lithotomy position.

2. The bladder is emptied and, if there is not epidural analgesia, the perineum is infiltrated or a pudendal nerve block produced.

3. When the breech is at the perineum the patient starts to bear down and an episiotomy is made where the perineum is distended.

4. With maternal effort the breech is delivered. If the legs are flexed they are delivered gently; if extended they can be flexed by pressure in the popliteal fossa to assist their delivery.

5. A towel is placed round the buttocks so that the obstetrician can support the fetal pelvis (grasping the abdomen may cause serious injury) while mother expels the trunk.

6. If the arms do not deliver spontaneously they can be flexed at the elbows and delivered. If the arms are extended the Løvset manoeuvre, Fig. 10.5, is used, rotating the fetus through 180° to bring the anterior shoulder below the pubis so that the arm can be brought down and delivered.

7. The baby is allowed to hang downward to assist flexion of the head. The hair line should appear below the pubis.

8. The feet and legs of the baby are lifted up and held by an assistant so that the head can be delivered by forceps, or by the Mauriceau–Smellie–Veit technique (the middle finger is placed in the baby's mouth to produce flexion, with the ring and index finger on the face beside the nose. With pressure on the occiput to increase flexion the head can be delivered by drawing the body down and then upwards).

Lack of oxygen during delivery is a major cause of mortality and morbidity, and delivery should not be delayed. The baby often passes meconium during delivery. The cord can be palpated to check for pulsation and fetal heart rate as soon as the pelvis is delivered. If there is need the baby can be delivered by breech extraction, using a combination of leg, groin and pelvic traction with forceps delivery of the head. In the hands of an expert this expedites delivery, but it is potentially more dangerous and traumatic than assisted delivery.

Fibroids in pregnancy

It is not uncommon for pregnant women to have fibroids and they do not usually cause problems. Fibroids may cause the uterus to appear large for dates, rarely they cause obstruction in labour or undergo red degeneration (see p. 188). Fibroids usually grow in pregnancy and become softer in consistency. It is not uncommon for a doctor or student to mistake a larger hard fibroid for a fetal head. They increases the risk of postpartum haemorrhage. Treatment is always conservative during pregnancy.

Ovarian tumours in pregnancy

These may be detected on examination early in pregnancy or by ultrasound; most are cysts. They may undergo torsion, haemorrhage or rupture, and can also obstruct labour. Because of the possibility of complications and the risk of malignancy (probably not more than 3 per cent) it is usual to remove cysts early in the second trimester, though many regress spontaneously before then.

Intrauterine death

Death of the fetus may occur during pregnancy or labour. In the latter case it is diagnosed quickly but in pregnancy the doctor may find that the fetal heart is undetectable. This may occur when neither he nor the patient had any suspicion of anything amiss or the patient may become suspicious because of lack of movements. In either event it is essential for the doctor or midwife to be absolutely certain of the death, before committing himself. Confirmation can be obtained from ultrasound, Doppler fetal heart detector or X-ray if necessary. A gentle and supportive explanation to the mother and father is required. Humanity indicates induction of labour as soon as this is safe and feasible. Everything possible should be done to make labour as easy as possible and staff should be encouraged to go and talk to the patient or couple, rather than staying away, as happens all too often.

It is in everybody's interest to know the reason for the death and the parents will usually consent to a post mortem examination and any other appropriate investigations. At the time only a limited explantation may be possible but it is vital to arrange for further interviews with obstetrician, paediatrician, genetic counsellor or other appropriate person so that the grief, guilt, anger, suspicion and other emotions, as well as the need for an explanation, can be satisfied. The counselling will include discussion of the future and risks involved in any future pregnancy.

It is important to remember and exclude the possibility of bleeding due to a maternal coagulation defect.

Prolonged pregnancy

By definition this is a pregnancy which has exceeded 42 weeks. Induction for postmaturity is a controversial subject and is bedevilled by the need to be sure of the dates. In most cases this is possible from the dates themselves, the usual menstrual cycle and clinical and ultrasound observations during pregnancy but it can still be difficult if: 1. the patient is not seen during the first half of pregnancy; 2. ultrasound is unavailable or 3. the fetus is larger or smaller than normal. After term the fetus is at greater risk both of disproportion, because of continued growth, and of asphyxia due to placental insufficiency. For this reason most obstetricians advise induction of labour, to prevent undue prolongation of pregnancy, which is welcomed by most women.

Further reading

Russell, J.K. (1981). Breech: vaginal delivery or caesarean section. *British Medical Journal* **285**, 830–1.

11

Medical disorders and pregnancy*

Anaemia

Anaemia is a common problem in pregnancy, particularly in countries and districts where nutrition is poor and antenatal care nonexistent. There is an increase in plasma volume (30 per cent) and red cell volume in pregnancy, but the former is greater and there is, therefore, a small decrease in haemoglobin concentration and in the packed cell volume. Haemoglobin of 10 g/100 ml blood is acceptable during the last trimester. In pregnancy additional iron is required for the fetus (400 mg), placenta (150 mg), mother (100 mg) to cover the increase in red cells. A variable amount of blood is lost at, and after delivery so the demands on the maternal iron stores may be considerable.

Iron deficiency anaemia

The commonest form of anaemia; it is diagnosed from microcytosis, low mean corpuscular haemoglobin concentration, low serum iron level and increased iron binding capacity. The anaemia may be precipitated by loss of blood for example due to haemorrhoids, hook worms or malaria.

Increased demands for folic acid in pregnancy can lead to megaloblastic anaemia which may occur on its own or with iron deficiency anaemia. The serum folate concentration is reduced, macrocytosis occurs and the bone marrow is megaloblastic. It is rare to find vitamin B12 deficiency, but wise to measure the serum vitamin B12 concentration, particularly in vegetarians.

Most obstetricians advise pregnant women to take iron and folic acid prophylactically during the second and third trimesters of pregnancy. In the first trimester it is best avoided because of the frequency of gastro-intestinal upset, which may be aggravated by iron which might be harmful (perhaps by reducing zinc absorption). The need to give prophylactic iron to women with normal haemoglobin levels, particularly in their first pregnancy is increasingly being questioned. When iron is given, it is usual to give it with folic acid, the demand for which is increased by multiple pregnancy and anti-convulsant therapy. A suitable dosage is 100 mg ferrous iron and 300 µg folic acid contained in one tablet daily.

*See Findlay, *Reproduction and the Fetus*, Chapter 6 (N.B. Table 6.2)

If there is iron deficiency, treatment is normally by oral iron and folic acid. If the haemoglobin is low and the pregnancy is well advanced, or if the patient cannot tolerate or take oral iron, intravenous iron (with iron dextran 50 mg/ml) is an alternative; caution is required as reactions can occur and oral iron should be given whenever possible. Intramuscular injections (iron dextran or iron sorbitol) can be also given but are painful and stain the skin. Folic acid deficiency is normally corrected by oral therapy, up to 1000 µg daily.

The Haemoglobinopathies

These should be diagnosed either from the history or by screening patients from appropriate parts of the globe at booking. Thalassaemia major is rarely associated with pregnancy while thalassaemia minor causes a less severe hypochromic microcytic anaemia, which does not have any specific effect on pregnancy.

Sickle cell anaemia

When the patient is homozygous for the sickle gene pregnancy is dangerous, quite apart from genetic considerations; the perinatal mortality is approximately 30 per cent. Anaemia increases during pregnancy and crises may occur, while there is an increased risk of intrauterine growth retardation and perinatal mortality. Iron or folate deficiency can occur, and the anaemia may be exacerbated by malaria. Iron deficiencies do not normally occur, treatment consists of the administration of folic acid and transfusion when necessary; expert supervision is essential. Exchange transfusion is currently under trial as a method of treatment. Sickle cell trait has little effect on maternal or perinatal mortality, though there is an increased incidence of urinary tract infection.

Heart disease

Rheumatic heart disease is less common than it was, and most patients have had acquired or congenital heart disease assessed or corrected by surgery before they become pregnant. In any case of suspected or known heart disease a cardiologist's advice should be obtained. The increased blood volume, body fluid, body weight, and cardiac output put an additional strain on the heart during pregnancy.

The chief complications and dangers are heart failure, endocarditis and thrombo-embolism. Patients with cardiomyopathy, pulmonary hypertension and Marfan's syndrome are at particular risk, and the dangers are greatly increased for those women who do not receive antenatal care. Patients on Warfarin are at increased risk of fetal abnormality during the first trimester (abnormalities of the facial bones and microcephaly have been reported), and of fetal and maternal haemorrhage during late pregnancy and labour. Balancing the risks can be difficult but a change to heparin in the last trimester is safer.

Management

Measures to prevent complications include close supervision by physician and obstetrician, adequate rest (if necessary in hospital), prompt treatment of infection and the use of diuretics and other therapy when required. Occasionally cardiac surgery is justified during pregnancy. In labour antibiotic cover by penicillin and gentamicin, or another aminoglycoside is given with appropriate treatment for the heart condition. Avoidance of undue stress in labour is achieved by adequate analgesia (expert advice is required particularly in relation to regional anaesthesia) and the use of forceps to shorten the second stage. Caution is required with intravenous fluids and oxytocics.

The use of a smaller dose of ergometrine and syntocinon than usual may be wise, but the complete omission of an oxytocic may lead to postpartum haemorrhage. After delivery supervision must continue. For those with significant disease it is important to ensure that there is adequate support to enable the woman to cope with her home commitments, without detriment to her health.

Diabetes mellitus

This disease in pregnancy is dangerous for mother and fetus. In addition to those who have diabetes before pregnancy, there is a condition of gestational diabetes where the glucose tolerance test is abnormal only in pregnancy. Potential diabetics are those in whom there are factors which make diabetes more likely, including:

1. Previous babies over 4.2 kg (9 lb).
2. Previous unexplained stillbirth or neonatal death.
3. Family history of diabetes.
4. Repeated glycosuria.
5. Polyhydramnios.
6. Recurrent infections.
7. Excessive weight.

If diabetes is suspected a glucose tolerance test is required to establish the diagnosis, but a random blood sugar test is helpful when there is glycosuria (which is often physiological) as a screening test. An abnormal result is most likely in the third trimester, but any patient likely to have diabetes must be investigated as early in pregnancy as possible.

The risks of diabetes in pregnancy for the mother include:

1. Progression of nephropathy, neuropathy and retinopathy.
2. Increased incidence of polyhydramnios, pre-eclampsia, premature labour and infection.
3. Hypoglycaemia and/or hyperglycaemia due to difficulty in controlling the disease.
4. The dangers of delivering a large baby.

For the fetus there is an increased risk of fetal abnormality, intrauterine death and macrosomia.

The neonate is at risk from prematurity, respiratory distress, traumatic delivery, hypoglycaemia and hyperbilirubinaemia.

Pregnancy Assessment and Counselling

Before pregnancy careful assessment of the dangers, counselling and meticulous (even obsessive) control of the disease is required. When the danger to the mother is high and the chance of successful pregnancy poor (e.g. with long standing diabetes, nephropathy and retinopathy), advice against pregnancy may be required and termination justified.

Management in Pregnancy

Pregnancy makes control of diabetes more difficult. There is an increased need for insulin, due to maternal levels of antagonists such as placental lactogen and steroids; while the demands of the fetus for glucose predispose the mother to hypoglycaemia and ketosis. It is clear that there is a direct relationship between the degree of control and the likelihood of complications such as fetal abnormality, macrosomia and polyhydramnios. Care should be shared between physician and obstetrician, who should see the patient, preferably together, at least every fortnight. Dietary control will be adequate for those with mild chemical diabetes, although all patients need revised advice, as in these guidelines:

1. An intake of 1500–2400 calories a day including 150–240 g of carbohydrate and 100 g of protein.

2. Oral hypoglycaemic agents are generally avoided in pregnancy and the insulin regime is usually a twice daily injection of soluble, longer acting insulin controlled by blood glucose levels.

3. Patients are admitted to hospital if there is any complication or if control is not satisfactory.

4. Home monitoring by women of their blood glucose levels to control their diabetes.

5. Maternal glycosylated haemoglobin (HbA_1) level indicates the efficiency of control over the preceding 6 weeks.

Delivery

In the past many diabetic mothers were delivered at 37–38 weeks by caesarean section. Now, however, close supervision and monitoring of fetal wellbeing, coupled with better diabetic control, enable more babies to be delivered vaginally, some at term. The timing and method of delivery depend on the diabetic control, the presence or absence of complications such as pre-eclampsia, and the size, health and maturity of the fetus. The majority of diabetic women are still delivered at about 38 weeks. Those with complications are delivered earlier and those with a good diabetic control later. No diabetic patient should continue a pregnancy beyond term.

The neonate will require expert paediatric care, particularly if it is premature, as hypoglycaemia is common. The mother will need much less insulin after delivery and careful supervision is required at this time. Intravenous glucose and insulin during labour and the immediate postpartum period give the best control.

Hypertension in pregnancy

Hypertension may have been diagnosed before pregnancy or in the antenatal clinic. If women are seen early in pregnancy it is easier to discriminate between hypertension associated with pregnancy (see pre-eclampsia) and that due to other causes. Pre-existing hypertension which may be essential, renal or due to rarer causes, such as coarctation of the aorta and phaeochromocytoma, increases the risk of pre-eclamptic hypertension. Maternal hypertension increases the risk of intrauterine growth retardation, perinatal loss, placental abruption and cerebo-vascular accident.

Management

With previously undiagnosed hypertension the patient should have an appropriate history, examination and investigation. If the blood pressure is greater than 140/90 it is usually best to admit her for investigation, which should include tests of renal function and measurement of urinary vanillyl mandelic acid to exclude phaeochromocytoma. Consultation with a physician may be advisable. With a systolic pressure above 150 or a diastolic above 100 treatment should be considered (Table 11.1).

These drugs have been introduced cautiously because of the fear of adverse fetal effects. Lowering the blood pressure to normal levels does not appear to harm the fetus.

Rest is an important part of the treatment and of the prevention of an increase in the blood pressure. Such patients should not work and admission to hospital may be necessary for observation, and adjustment of treatment when blood pressure is over 140/90. Patients should be seen frequently for blood pressure checks and close supervision of the pregnancy to detect, in particular, any hypertension or fetal hazard. Diuretics and sedatives are not normally helpful in treating essential hypertension and should be avoided.

Table 11.1 Drugs used to treat hypertension during pregnancy.

Drug	Action	Dose
Methyldopa	Probably central adreno-ceptor block by methylnoradrenaline	250–750 mg orally thrice daily
Labetalol	Adrenoceptor block peripherally) block (cardiac)	200–800 mg orally 100–300 mg orally thrice daily
Hydralazine	Arteriolar dilatation	25–75 mg orally twice daily

Early induction and delivery may be required depending on the health of mother and fetus. Ergometrine is best avoided in the third stage because of its hypertensive effect. A lecithin-sphingomyelin ratio in liquor greater than 2:1 indicates adaquate surfactant, therefore RDS is unlikely.

Thyroid disease

There is an increase in thyroid binding globulin in pregnancy which means that levels of hormones found are higher. The levels of free tri-iodothyronine, thyroxine and TSH are, however, unaffected and can therefore be used as measures of thyroid function. Hyperthyroidism can be treated with carbimazole, propylthiouracil or surgery, the use of radioactive iodine being contraindicated. Occasionally the use of antithyroid drugs will cause fetal goitre; these drugs are excreted in milk and mothers taking them should not breast-feed. Hypothyroidism is treated with thyroxine and there is no contraindication to breast-feeding.

Table 11.2 Serious effects on embryo or fetus of maternal infection.

Infection	Main danger	Abnormalities in the neonate
Chlamydia	3rd Trimester	Neonatal pneumonia and ophthalmitis
Cytomegalovirus (CMV)	1st, 2nd Trimester	Microcephaly, hydrocephalus, mental retardation, deafness, choroido-retinitis, anaemia, pneumonia
Gonorrhoea	3rd Trimester	Neonatal ophthalmitis
Vaginal Herpes	3rd Trimester	Neonatal infection
Malaria	1st, 3rd Trimester	Low birth weight
Rubella	1st Trimester	Eye (cataract, retinitis, glaucoma) deafness, congenital heart defects, approximately 33% in 1st month, 25% in second, 10% in third
	2nd, 3rd Trimester	Small for dates, microcephaly, hepatosplenomegaly, thrombo-cytopenia. Infections at and after birth
Syphilis	1st, 2nd Trimester	Hydrocephalus, mental retardation, deafness, bone (including nose) neurological, Hutchinson's teeth
Toxoplasmosis	1st, 2nd Trimester	Microcephaly, hydrocephalus, microphthalmia, choroidoretinitis, cerebral calcification
Varicella	1st, 2nd Trimester	Cortical atrophy, choroidoretinitis, cataract, scarring of skin, limb hypoplasia, rudimentary digits, muscular atrophy

Thromboembolic disease

Thromboembolic disease in pregnancy is not uncommon and remains a significant cause of maternal death. The investigations are the same as for non-pregnant patients. Superficial venous thrombosis is treated by local therapy, rest, bandaging and elevation of the legs.

Deep venous thrombosis and pulmonary embolism is treated by heparin anticoagulation, starting with an intravenous loading dose of 5000 units followed by a continuous intravenous infusion of heparin 40 000 units per 24 hours.

A less satisfactory alternative is to give the heparin, 10 000 units intravenously every 6 hours. Heparin does not cross the placenta, has a short life and its action can be reversed with protamine sulphate. It is convenient to switch to oral warfarin after 2–7 days, but warfarin does cross the placenta and should not be used in the first trimester when it may produce fetal optic atrophy and hypoplasia of the nasal bones. It is also contraindicated after 37 weeks because of the likelihood of labour. The action of warfarin can be reversed by giving vitamin K (phytomenadione) 10–20 mg intravenously or orally, or by fresh plasma. After 37 weeks heparin therapy is resumed. Heparin can be given subcutaneously, 5000 units every 4–6 hours and some patients can administer the drug themselves (in which case they can continue on heparin throughout pregnancy). Breast feeding is not contraindicated if the mother is being treated with heparin or warfarin.

Table 11.3 Some drugs which may harm the embryo or fetus.

Drug	Time	Possible effects
Alcohol	Throughout pregnancy	Fetal alcohol syndrome: growth retardation, withdrawal syndrome at birth, mental retardation, congenital heart disease, musculoskeletal defects, facial dysmorpho-genesis, minor genital defects (occurs in approximately 1 out of every 3 heavy drinkers)
Aminoglycosides	Throughout	Nephrotoxic, ototoxic
Androgens	Throughout	Masculinize the female
Antiprostaglandins		Premature closure of ductus arteriosus
Anti-thyroid	Throughout	Goitre
Chloramphenicol	Late	'Grey baby syndrome' in neonate
Corticosteroids	Late	Neonatal adrenal depression
Cytotoxic	Throughout	Growth retardation, facial abnormalities
Lithium		Goitre, cardiac abnormalities
Nicotine	Throughout	Low birth weight
Nitrofurantoin	Late	Hyperbilirubinamia
Podophyllin	Early	CNS effects
Progestogens	1st, 2nd Trimester	Masculinization of female
Stilboestrol	Early	Vaginal adenosis, later clear cell carcinoma
Streptomycin	Any	8th nerve damage
Sulphonamides	Late	Hyperbilirubinaemia, kernicterus
Tetracycline		Deposited in bone and teeth (which are discoloured)

Note. Any depressant drug (e.g. morphine sulphate, pethidine, magnesium sulphate, promethazine, antihistamines and benzodiazepines) given shortly before delivery may cause neonatal depression.
   Any drug of addiction taken in excess by the mother late in pregnancy may lead to withdrawal symptoms in the neonate.

Rhesus factor

A rhesus negative woman may produce anti-D antibodies against rhesus positive cells from a fetus either at abortion, delivery, amniocentesis, ectopic pregnancy or external version. She may also be sensitized by a rhesus positive blood transfusion. Antibodies (IgG) formed in this way cross the placenta and haemolyse fetal red cells causing anaemia and jaundice after delivery (when the fetal liver is unable to cope with the haemolysis). The disease is becoming rare due to prevention (see p. 79, 96) but cases still occur either because anti-D was not given or because the haemorrhage was larger than usual or occured during the course of pregnancy. The severity tends to increase with successive pregnancies but if the husband is heterozygous there is a 50 per cent chance that the fetus will be rhesus negative and therefore unaffected. ABO incompatibility is also protective.

Rhesus antibody levels or titres are measured at booking, 28 and 34 weeks. If there are antibodies, the tests are repeated regularly and if the levels are rising or moderately high and the baby may be affected, amniocentesis is carried out and the optical density at 450 nm (bile pigment) is calculated and plotted on a Liley or other chart which shows zones indicating the severity of the disease. With severe disease, the fetus becomes hydropic (with ascites, gross oedema) and then dies. In severe cases transuterine intraperitoneal transfusion of rhesus negative blood may be given from 24 weeks. After 34 weeks early delivery may be required with appropriate treatment of the baby if necessary (see p. 65).

Maternal infections

These will affect the baby, and those liable to produce serious abnormalities are included in Table 11.2.

Other problems

Almost any medical, surgical or psychiatric condition can occur in association with pregnancy. Cooperation and consultation between the obstetrician and others involved in the patient's care will enable the woman to receive the best advice and treatment. This may include termination when the pregnancy is likely to affect the mother's health or prevent treatment (e.g. of malignant disease), or where the disease is so severe that there is no realistic prospect of delivery of a live child (e.g. severe nephritis). Almost all drugs (not heparin) reach the fetus and while few are known to have adverse effects none should be administered to a woman who is known to be pregnant or may be pregnant, unless there is a strong indication and the risk to the fetus has been evaluated. (See Table 11.3).

Further reading

Lewis, Peter Ed. (1983). *Clinical Pharmacology in Obstetrics*. Wright, Bristol.
Coid, C.R.Ed. (1977). *Infections and Pregnancy*. Academic Press, London.

12

The complications of labour

Preterm labour

Labour starting before the 37th week.
  Causes of preterm labour:

1. Cervical incompetence
2. Congenital uterine abnormality
3. Premature rupture of the membranes
4. Antepartum haemorrhage (usually placental abruption)
5. Polyhydramnios
6. Multiple pregnancy
7. Fetal abnormality
8. Intrauterine death
9. Maternal pyrexia or illness
10. Trauma
11. Intrauterine growth retardation

The patient should be admitted as speedily as possible; if the pregnancy is less than 34 weeks she should be admitted to a hospital with a neonatal intensive care unit. In many cases there is a reason for the onset of labour and it may be inappropriate to oppose it. Generally, however, if the gestation time is less than 35 or 36 weeks and the fetus and pregnancy appear otherwise normal, an attempt is made to halt labour. It is important to assess the strength of contractions and to assess the state of the cervix since some patients have painful contractions without starting labour.

Treatment

Ethyl alcohol has been used for this purpose but the β-sympathomimetic drugs; notably salbutamol and ritodrine, are the most popular at present. The chosen drug is given by intravenous infusion, increasing the dose until the contractions have stopped, then continuing for a period of 11 hours before switching to intramuscular or oral therapy. Prostaglandin synthetase inhibitors are contraindicated because of their association with closure of the ductus arteriosus.

These drugs should not be used if there is antepartum haemorrhage, hypertension or heart disease. Pulmonary oedema is a possible complication and pulmonary hypertension may occur if the patient is also taking steroids. Sometimes these drugs are used to delay labour while dexamethasone 4 mg 8-hourly by intramuscular injection or another glucocorticoid is given to induce the production of pulmonary surfactant and reduce the risk of the respiratory distress syndrome (see p. 49). Careful observation of the mother, notably the pulse and fetal heart rate every 5 minutes while the dose is increasing, is mandatory. The maternal pulse should not exceed 140 per minute.

Ritodrine HCI is given in a solution of 500 ml 5 per cent dextrose (50 mg). The drip is started at 50 μg/minute, increasing by 50 μg every 10 minutes until the uterus is controlled. In higher doses it is wise to use a more concentrated solution;

1. 100 mg/500 ml 5 per cent dextrose when dose exceeds 200μg/minute
2. 200 mg/500 ml 5 per cent dextrose when dose exceeds 400μg/minute

Oral ritodrine is given in a dose of 10 mg 2–6 hourly as long as required.

If pre-term delivery occurs, epidural anaesthesia is preferable to pethidine or general anaesthesia because there is less fetal depression, and caesarean section is safer for the very premature small babies. Vaginal delivery of pre-term babies should be particularly gentle, facilitated if necessary by episiotomy and forceps for those between 2.0 and 2.5 kg.

Premature rupture of the membranes

This is often unexplained but may occur with multiple pregnancy, polyhydramnios, trauma, cervical incompetence, malpresentation or amnionitis (infection of the amnion). Labour may follow and there is a danger of ascending infection (greatly increased if there is vaginal interference). The cord may prolapse at any time.

The patient should be admitted to hospital and be nursed in bed. After the history and general examination, a vaginal examination should normally be carried out (this should be done by an experienced obstetrician using a sterile technique). The state of the cervix should be checked and the presence of the cord excluded if the presenting part is not an engaged head. It is sensible to take a high vaginal swab for culture. Early in the third trimester vaginal examination may be deferred to reduce the risk of infection. In some cases the membranes have not ruptured and urine and vaginal discharge are the cause of alarm.

After 35 weeks there is no advantage in delaying labour and there is a risk of infection. Before, it may be justifiable to attempt to delay labour with rest and ritodrine or salbutamol given prophylactically (see Preterm labour, p. 125). Occasionally it is the hind waters (the liquor above the presenting part) which leak. It is not unknown for ruptured membranes to stop leaking, in which case the patient may be mobilized.

Abnormalities in the first stage

Abnormal uterine action

The uterus may contract normally or the contractions may be weak (hypotonic), excessive (hypertonic) or unco-ordinated. In hypotonic uterine action the contractions are typically short, weak, infrequent and irregular. This behaviour occurs quite often in primigravid patients for no obvious reason but it may also be a response to cephalopelvic disproportion. The opposite state of hypertonic action may be produced by injudicious administration of oxytocin, but can also occur spontaneously or, in a multigravida, in the presence of obstruction. Hypotonic inertia causes slow progress in labour, maternal fatigue and loss of morale and dehydration. Hypertonic action may result in a quick labour but is painful and exhausting for the mother, can lead to uterine rupture or amniotic embolism, and may cause fetal hypoxia. With inco-ordinate action the contractions are variable in strength, irregular in time and may not start at the fundus (as is normal), or may spread asymetrically. The mother suffers the distress of contractions and slow progress, while the contractions may also cause fetal hypoxia if they are hypertonic.

Less common than abnormality of uterine action is cervical dystocia when the cervix does not dilate; this may be idiopathic or secondary to cervical surgery.

In the presence of hydramnios, multiple pregnancy, malposition of the head (particularly occipitoposterior), obstruction (in a primagravida) or malpresentation the uterus tends to act less efficiently and labour is often prolonged.

Long labour

In days gone by many women endured labours of 48 hours or even more, but nowadays most obstetricians believe that labour should not last longer than twelve hours in a primigravid patient. The aspects to be considered during labour are:

1. Is labour progressing? (judged by the contractions, descent of the presenting part, cervical dilation)
2. Is there fetal distress? (judged by fetal heart rate monitoring, fetal blood sampling)
3. Is there maternal distress? (judged by the mother or observation of her)

Lack of progress

If labour is not progressing because of disproportion, caesarean section is required. If the lack of progress is due to hypotonic uterine action, rupture of the membranes, if required, together with intravenous oxytocin should have the necessary 'accelerating' effect. Great caution is required in giving oxytocin to multigravid women as it can readily produce hypertonic action with risk to mother and fetus. It is important to remember that a full bladder may inhibit uterine contraction at any stage of labour. Maternal distress can be relieved by caring staff, analgesics (particularly epidural anaesthesia), and fluid replacement; the last of these often appears to have a beneficial effect on uterine action as well.

When labour is not progressing as it should the cause should be identified, particularly disproportion (see p. 134), as well as any deficiencies in treatment such as failure to correct dehydration. Long labour and poor progress are worrying and exhausting for the patient; she needs additional explanation, encouragement and support as a result.

A contraction ring occurs very rarely nowadays. It occurs in a prolonged labour when there is a tight ring due to muscle spasm, usually at the level of the fetal neck. It can be felt abdominally and is associated with lack of progress. It can also cause retention of the placenta.

Abnormalities in the second stage

It used to be the rule that the second stage should not normally last longer than one hour for a primigravida and 30 minutes for a multigravida. It is now recognized that there is advantage in waiting, when the cervix is fully dilated, until the patient is ready to push. Provided that the fetus is in good condition this is not harmful. These times are guidelines for pushing and any decision to intervene depends on the mother's feelings, her general state and that of the fetus, the degree of progress and the prospects of ultimate spontaneous delivery.

Causes of delay

These are similar to those in the first stage. Abnormal uterine action is likely to continue in the second stage, and after a long or difficult labour the mother may not have sufficient energy to 'push' effectively. An occipitoposterior position or face presentation is more likely to progress slowly. If there is disproportion progress will cease.

Deep transverse arrest

This occurs when the fetal head reaches the level of the ischial spines in the transverse position. The head may have descended in the transverse position or there may have been partial rotation from an original occipitoposterior position. Because the head, which is deflexed, cannot rotate and there is insufficient space for the head to descend, further labour is effectively obstructed. Further progress, or forceps delivery, can only take place if the head is rotated to the occipito-anterior or posterior position (the latter is less favourable because of possible incomplete flexion and the larger diameters, at engagement and delivery).

Face presentation and obstruction of labour

The head is completely extended in face presentation. If it is mento-anterior (the chin anterior) the head can flex and is delivered if this happens. If it is mento-posterior, however, the head which is already fully extended cannot flex because it is against the sacrum and coccyx so that delivery is not possible.

If the head is too large for the pelvis or there is brow presentation labour is also obstructed (as it is in deep transverse arrest).

General management

If there is no progress the reason should be assessed and delivery expedited.

The urgency will depend on the presence or absence of fetal distress and the degree of maternal distress. If the delay is at the perineum an episiotomy may be all that is required. Above this level forceps or ventouse must be chosen, and can be used to correct a transverse or posterior position, if necessary, before proceeding to delivery. Alternatively the position can be corrected manually. If there is disproportion caesarean section is the safest course; if there is doubt about this a trial of forceps can be performed in theatre with everyone prepared to proceed to caesarean section should it be necessary. Postpartum haemorrhage is more likely after a long labour, particularly if it has been characterized by hypotonic or inco-ordinate uterine action.

Shoulder Dystocia

One of the most alarming situations in obstetrics occurs when, having delivered the head, the obstetrician is unable to deliver the shoulders. Excessive traction from below may result in trauma to the baby (Erb's palsy, C.5,6 or Klumpke's C.7,8.), while delay in excess of 5 minutes is likely to cause asphyxia, since the baby cannot breathe and the cord may be occluded. Additionally venous return from head and neck to the heart is often obstructed.

This is most likely to occur with large babies but may occur as a result of failure of rotation of the shoulders or because of a tumour or abnormality. Where possible the situation should be anticipated and caesearean section undertaken or an experienced obstetrician should attend the delivery. When in difficulty the rotation of the head should be checked to see if the shoulders have rotated (the head may be rotated in the wrong direction). With correct rotation of the head and traction posteriorly, the anterior shoulder should come down and be delivered. Fundal pressure or assistance with rotation abdominally will often enable delivery to be completed. Otherwise the operator can attempt to rotate the shoulders digitally from below. Cleidotomy (cutting the clavicle) or bringing an arm down may be solutions for an experienced obstetrician when the patient is anaesthetised, but if these measures are needed the baby may well have died and there is a high risk of trauma, including vaginal laceration, extension of episiotomy and uterine rupture.

Rapid labour

Some mothers labour much more efficiently and rapidly than average, and in some multigravidae labour may last approximately an hour and the second stage consist of only a few contractions. A first labour of under 6 hours should be noted since the next may be very rapid. Some labours are completed in under an hour and such deliveries are described as precipitate. The risk is that the mother will deliver before she can get to hospital or receive professional assistance. All may be well but there is a risk to the baby and the prospect is worrying for everyone concerned. It is sensible therefore to discuss the advisability of admission to hospital just before term and possible induction when a short labour seems likely.

Fetal distress

This is a state in which the wellbeing of the fetus is affected by lack of oxygen or nutrition. The growth-retarded fetus is at greatest risk and will be affected quicker than the normal, full-term fetus. Evidence of fetal distress can be obtained from the fetal heart rate, the fetal electrocardiogram, amniotic fluid and the fetal blood pH.

Fetal heart rate

This can be counted by the Pinard stethoscope applied to the mother's abdomen, an electrode applied to the fetal scalp or buttock or a transducer using the Doppler principle on the mother's abdomen.

From a transducer or electrode the impulses are fed into a fetal heart monitor which measures the interval between beats and displays the rate, so that variations are shown clearly on the recording. These should normally be related to a trace of uterine contractions obtained through a pressure transducer on the abdomen or a catheter inserted into the uterus.

Signs of fetal distress are:

1. Fetal tachycardia (rate exceeds 160 per minute).
2. Fetal bradycardia (rate less than 120 per minute).
3. Lack of beat to beat variation (see Fig. 12.1).
4. Late decelerations (Type II see Fig. 12.2).
5. Early decelerations (Type I see Fig. 12.3).

In general tachycardia occurs before bradycardia. When Type I decelerations are seen this may be due to head compression, but Type II decelerations may follow if there is hypoxia. Transient bradycardia is not infrequent at the onset of epidural anaesthesia and in the second stage. The interpretation of these and other signs requires experience, and consideration of the other information available about the health of mother, fetus and progress of labour. For example, maternal pyrexia or tachycardia will affect the fetal heart rate. If there is evidence of fetal distress the mother should change from the supine position, if she is in it, to a lateral position and oxygen can be given by face mask while the situation is assessed.

Meconium

This is often passed by the fetus when distressed and can be seen in the liquor if the membranes are ruptured. It is important to distinguish between fresh (green) and old (darker) meconium. Aspiration of meconium by the fetus is liable to occur and complicates respiration post partum (see p. 54).

Fetal blood pH

Blood from the scalp or buttock can be obtained using an amnioscope. The normal pH is 7.35 and less than 7.20 is abnormal. Values close to 7.20 merit close observation of the fetus and repetition of the examination after a short interval. To be of value, pH measurements must be obtained speedily and accurately, or they will do more harm than good. If there is maternal acidosis

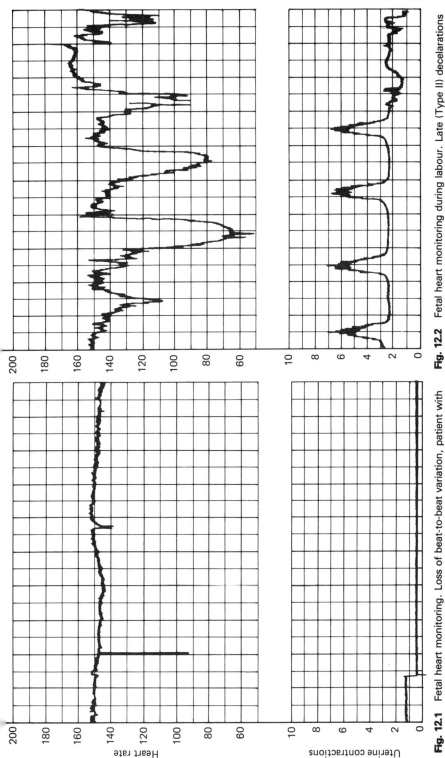

Fig. 12.1 Fetal heart monitoring. Loss of beat-to-beat variation, patient with pre-eclampsia and fetal growth retardation.

Fig. 12.2 Fetal heart monitoring during labour. Late (Type II) decelerations occuring after contractions.

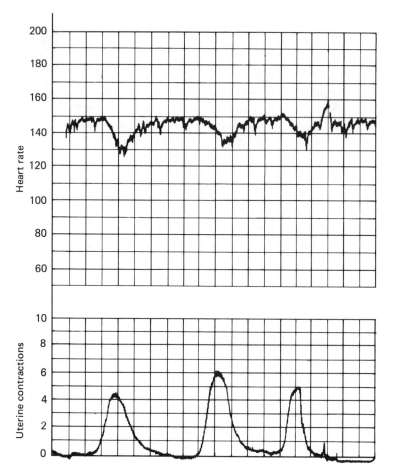

Fig. 12.3　Fetal heart monitoring during labour. Early (Type II) declarations occuring with contraction, this is not abnormal.

there is maternal acidosis this will affect the fetal pH; caution is then required in interpreting results unless the pH of the mother and fetus are available.

Action

If there is fetal distress action is required to expedite delivery. Appropriate treatment will vary from caesarean section to delivery by forceps, ventouse or episiotomy. Fetal distress will be more likely to occur when there is growth retardation, maternal hypertension or diabetes, multiple pregnancy or antepartum haemorrhage. In these cases, as well as those of elderly primigravidae and women with bad obstetric histories, the patient should be advised to have the benefits of fetal monitoring. Monitoring is no substitute for observation of the patient however, and concentration on monitors, equipment failure and misinterpretation of results can cause staff to miss or ignore important signs and symptoms and make wrong decisions.

Prolapse of the cord and cord presentation

Prolapse of the cord means that the cord lies beside or below the presenting part after rupture of the membranes. This is likely when the presenting part is not engaged or does not fit well in the pelvis, e.g. with a flexed breech. It may be discovered accidentally on vaginal examination, be visible outside the vulva, or be suspected because fetal distress occurs.

The patient should be placed in the left lateral position (Sim's position is best) and the bed or trolley tipped head down (Fig. 12.4). The presenting part is pushed up by the fingers to relieve pressure on the cord. If the trolley cannot be tipped the patient may be placed in the knee-elbow position and the presenting part pushed up as described above. This position and the pressure should be maintained until delivery is imminent. There is no point in attempting to replace the cord above the presenting part but it should be kept within the vagina as drying and a lower temperature when it is outside can

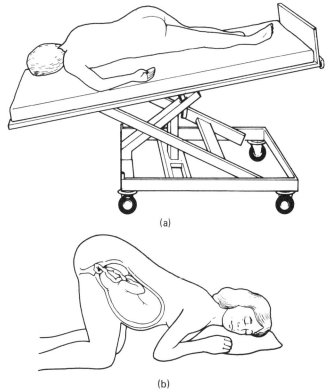

(a)

(b)

Fig. 12.4 Correction of a prolapsed cord using; (a) Sim's position on a tilted trolley; or (b) as an alternative, the genu-pectoral position.

cause spasm of the vessels. Pulsation of the cord vessels should be felt unless the cord is compressed or the fetus dead.

Cord presentation may be felt through the membranes at vaginal examination. The membranes should not be ruptured and caesearean section may be indicated.

Cephalo-pelvic disproportion

The importance of recognizing disproportion has already been emphasized. Failure to do so can lead to long, unhappy labours, uterine infections and rupture, fetal hypoxia, death and trauma. The strikingly small pelvis or large fetus should be detected during pregnancy. If the fetal head does not engage in a cephalic presentation the obstetrician should discover in the last week or two before term whether it will go through the pelvic brim on standing or if pushed down by the examiner.

If the fetal head does not go in and no explanation is evident a trial of labour may be the best way to manage the situation. This is appropriate when the head is presenting and the outcome of labour is in doubt because of possible disproportion. Trial of labour means that there is suspected disproportion and the progress of labour is closely watched by an experienced obstetrician; if it does not occur satisfactorily, caesarean section should be undertaken. There is no place for trial of labour in breech presentation or where there is a major degree of disproportion.

X-ray Pelvimetry
This is much less used than formerly because of the desire to avoid irradiation and the poor correlation between radiological forecasts and the actual outcome of labour. It is helpful with breech presentation, and after caesarean section to assess the chance of vaginal delivery in a subsequent pregnancy.

Unexpected disproportion
During labour doctors and midwives should always be alert to the possibility of disproportion which can occur unexpectedly in any woman, for example with a brow presentation or a baby larger than she has had before. Neglect will lead to obstructed labour, and in the presence of continuing contraction, to a ruptured uterus.

Complications in the third stage

If part or all of the placenta is retained in the uterus, it should be removed because of the risk of postpartum haemorrhage. If delivery has not occurred within 20 minutes of delivery action is required. Sometimes the placenta is retained when there is retention of urine and catheterization will solve both problems. In hospital a drip should be set up and blood sent for cross matching; outside a fully equipped maternity unit (the 'flying squad') should be summoned. The placenta may be removed under epidural anaesthesia (if already induced), general anaesthesia or pudendal nerve block. In the rare case when the placenta is abnormally adherent and there is no bleeding it may be safest to leave it (placenta accreta, see p. 139).

Inversion of the uterus

This results from cord traction when the placenta is still attached and the uterus relaxed. If it happens the uterus can usually easily be replaced immediately. This becomes more difficult if there is delay when shock and haemorrhage may occur. An experienced obstetrician can usually restore the position after removing the placenta with the aid of an anaesthetic.

Post partum haemorrhage

This is defined as the loss of 500 ml or more within 24 hours of delivery. Measurement of blood loss is difficult and the amount is generally underestimated. Most haemorrhages occur soon after delivery; when they occur later, they are usually due to relaxation of the uterus or retained placental tissue.

The causes of postpartum haemorrhage (PPH) include:

1. Retained placenta.
2. Failure of the uterus to contract or remain contracted.
3. Vaginal, cervical or uterine trauma.
4. Coagulation disorders.

It is more likely to happen in those who have suffered a previous PPH, those with hydramnios, multiple pregnancy, hypotonic uterine action, fibroids, and conditions leading to coagulation defects.

Help should be obtained as speedily as possible (obstetrician, anaesthetist or 'flying squad') and the patient must not be left. An intravenous infusion should be started and blood sent for cross matching. If the uterus is relaxed it may be possible to stimulate a contraction by massaging the uterus or to produce one by intravenous ergometrine (10.5 mg) or a continuous syntocinon infusion. Bimanual compression is also effective but it is hard work. The bladder must be emptied and if necessary examination under anaesthetic may be required to exclude or repair vaginal or cervical lacerations, and to explore the uterus for retained tissue or rupture. If it is known that the placenta is incomplete the uterus must be explored as speedily as possible. Occasionally hysterectomy will be required to control haemorrhage but it is particularly important to exclude coagulation disorders before proceeding to surgery.

Coagulation disorders

These may occur after intrauterine death with retention of the fetus or placental absorption. They may follow an amniotic embolism or be a manifestation of a disease such as leukaemia or thrombocytopenic purpura. If suspected, a sample of blood should be observed in a glass tube where it should clot within 5–8 minutes. If possible a haematologist should be consulted; otherwise fresh blood and fresh frozen plasma should be given on the assumption that there is a deficiency of fibrinogen until the situation is controlled or the defect identified.

Ruptured uterus

This disaster usually occurs in labour in women who have previously had a caesarean section or hysterotomy. Rarely it occurs at the site of a myomectomy scar or uterine perforation. Any patient with a uterine scar should be assessed during pregnancy in relation to the risk of rupture so that she can be advised whether to have an elective caesarean section or a 'trial of scar' (a labour in which progress is monitored closely and caesarean section used if there is any problem). Rupture may occur in obstructed labour or rarely spontaneously in a multigravid patient. The signs may be 1. dramatic with pain, bleeding, and shock, or 2. less obvious with arrest of labour, pain, interpartum bleeding or postpartum haemorrhage.

Further reading

Chiswick, M.L. Ed. (1983). *Recent Advances in Perinatal Medicine — 1.* Churchill Livingstone, Edinburgh.

Lamont, R.F., Dunlop, D.P.H., Crawley, P. and Elder, M.G. (1983). Spontaneous Preterm Labour and Delivery at Under 34 Weeks Gestation. *British Medical Journal* i, 454–7.

13

Obstetric operations

Caesarean section

To the layman this may seem an easy and safe way for a baby to be born. In fact, it necessitates exposure of mother and fetus to a general or epidural anaesthetic, and the risk to the mother is greater than that of normal delivery. It is a major operation which exposes the mother to an increased risk of sepsis and thromboembolism, after which she must go home to look after a baby rather than to convalesce. Furthermore the uterine scar is a potential site of rupture in any future pregnancy. Nowadays, except in very rare circumstances, caesarean section is performed with a transverse incision through the lower segment which is thin and less likely to rupture in a subsequent pregnancy than the 'classical' vertical upper segment incision.

Indications for the operation include:

1. Fetal distress before or in the first stage of labour.
2. Intrauterine growth retardation (early in the 3rd trimester).
3. Multiple pregnancy (triplets or more).
4. Antepartum haemorrhage (placenta praevia, abruptio placentae).
5. Malposition and malpresentation.
6. Small premature babies.
7. Cephalopelvic disproportion.
8. Lack of progress in labour.
9. Previous caesarean section or uterine operation.
10. Medical disorders e.g. hypertension, previous subarachnoid haemorrhage.

Most of these are relative indications, agreed absolute indications include: two previous caesarean sections, cephalopelvic disproportion, placenta praevia types II–IV, fetal distress in the first stage and quadruplets.

Complications

Possible complications include; urinary, uterine and wound infection, retention of urine, paralytic ileus, haemorrhage, wound and uterine scar dehiscence, venous thrombosis and pulmonary embolism, as well as any complications attributable to anaesthesia. The bladder can be damaged, thus it is important to empty it before the operation. Infection in the uterine wound may interfere with healing and increase the risk of subsequent rupture.

The patient should be out of bed the day after operation, and able to go home within 10 days.

Forceps delivery

These have been used to assist delivery for over 300 years. They can be used to deliver the baby, control delivery, or to correct the position or presentation of the fetus. Most forceps are designed only for traction or control (e.g. Neville Barnes, Milne Murray, Wrigley's) but Kielland's forceps can be used for rotation (Fig. 13.1).

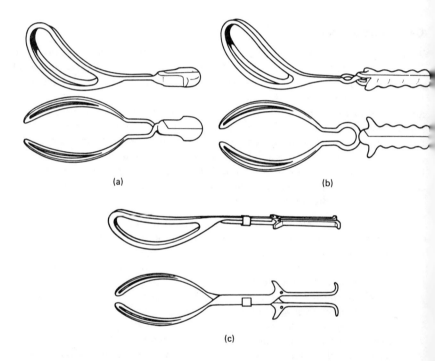

(a)

(b)

(c)

Fig. 13.1   Forceps: (a) Wrigley's (low cavity) forceps (b) forceps for low or mid cavity and (c) Kielland's forceps.

Forceps delivery should not be undertaken unless:

1. There is an adequate indication.
2. The patient is in the second stage of labour.
3. The head is at or below the level of the ischial spines.

4. The position of the head has been identified.
5. The bladder is empty.
6. There is no disproportion.
7. The uterus is contracting.

Attempts at forceps delivery before full dilatation of the cervix, with a high head or disproportion are unlikely to succeed. If attempted, this may result in severe trauma to the mother and baby.

Analgesia is essential and can be obtained either by general anaesthesia, or by epidural or pudendal nerve block (with infiltration of the vulva).

It is not possible to achieve delivery by traction when the presentation is brow, face (mentoposterior position) or vertex in the transverse position. It may be possible to rotate any of these manually or with Kiellands's forceps (though considerable training and experience is required to use these instruments safely). When the head is in the occipitoposterior position it should be corrected though sometimes, if it is low in the pelvic cavity, it is justifiable to deliver it without rotation. Failure to follow the rules for the use of forceps can lead to fetal death or injury (e.g. cerebral damage, intracranial haemorrhage, facial nerve palsy and facial lacerations) and injury to the mother's genital tract (notably cervical and vaginal tears and fistulae) as well as postpartum haemorrhage.

Indications for forceps delivery

1. The need to shorten the second stage because of the mother's health (for example, cardiac disease, hypertension, previous cerebrovascular accident).
2. Fetal distress.
3. Maternal distress.
4. Delay in the second stage or failure to progress (more likely with malpresentation, e.g. face, or malposition such as occipito-transverse).
5. To control delivery of the head in breech, or occasionally preterm delivery.

Manual removal of the placenta

This is performed under regional or general anaesthesia as a sterile procedure. An intravenous infusion should be running and blood should be cross matched. The indication is retention of all, or part of the placenta within the uterus, or the need to exclude the latter. The hand is introduced through the cervix with the fingers straight and crowded together. The placental edge is found and using the other hand on the abdomen to exert counter pressure the placenta is separated from the uterus. Force is not required and the placenta should separate easily unless there is placenta accreta, (a rare condition where the placenta is adherent to the myometrium). After removal of the placenta the uterus should be checked to ensure that it is empty and there is no injury.

The ventouse

This comprises a cup which can be attached to the fetal head, a chain for traction and a vacuum flask and pump connected to the cup. The instrument can be used to deliver a fetus by traction or for rotation, and it is possible to apply it before the cervix is fully dilated. The appropriate sized cup is chosen from the sizes 30 mm, 40 mm and 50 mm and is applied to the scalp as near the occiput as possible.

Initially a vacuum of 0.2 kg/cm^2 is produced, this is increased to 0.8 kg/cm^2, over a period of 5–6 minutes, if the application is satisfactory. Traction can then be applied using the chain. The indications for use of the ventouse are similar to those of forceps but its use varies widely; some obstetricians use it often in preference to forceps, while others never use it at all. Little or no anaesthesia may be required, but the application and delivery can take longer than with forceps.

The cup may produce a cephalhaematoma (a collection of blood beneath the periosteum). Occasionally there are problems with the apparatus, the cup may come off the fetal head if it is not properly applied or if there is excessive traction.

There are other operations which are performed in obstetrics. Some of these such as amniocentesis have been described elsewhere, others, such as the destructive operations for dead or abnormal fetuses, are rarely performed. Further knowledge of these practical procedures can be gained by observation of them and by reference to operative textbooks.

Further reading

Myerscough, P.R. (1982). *Munro Kerr's Operative Obstetrics*. Baillière Tindall, London.

14

The healthy woman

Most women who seek gynaecological advice are not ill and many need only reassurance. It is not always easy, however, to define what is normal in relation to menstruation or what variations are acceptable.* The normal menstrual cycle is always quoted as 28 days, but few women always have 28 day cycles, and variation between 21 and 35 days is acceptable as normal, though the variable cycle may be tiresome because it is unpredictable.

Short cycles may be a nuisance because of their frequency, though it is not always clear whether each bleed is in fact a period. Longer and more variable cycles, such as 28–42 days or more, are often a source of concern to women or adolescents and to their relatives. These cycles are more likely to be anovulatory and contribute to infertility but do not usually signal anything seriously wrong. The more infrequent the periods the more justification there is for investigation and a spell of 6 months without a period is classified as amenorrhea (see p. 166) and should be investigated. The normal length of a period is from 1–7 days, usually 4 or 5.

The blood loss averages 30–40 ml but also varies considerably; if it exceeds 80 ml it is abnormal. A scanty loss does not mean that anything is wrong, but heavy periods (menorrhagia) may indicate disease. Mennorrhagia requires investigation and treatment because of the possible underlying pathology, the risk of anaemia, malaise and the inconvenience and embarrassment which may result. Clearly the patient's view of what happens is the important one, and it is not helpful to dismiss a woman's complaint of heavy periods on the grounds that she is not anaemic and/or that no abnormality has been found in the pelvis. Bleeding for longer than 7 days is not acceptable to most people, and sometimes it is difficult to distinguish between a long period and intermenstrual bleeding. Bleeding between periods is always abnormal except when it occurs briefly at midcycle, associated with ovulation.

Discharge can be equally difficult to assess and gynaecologists see women complaining of discharge who appear normal on examination, while others with an abnormal discharge deny having such symptoms. All women have a little discharge derived from cervical mucus, vaginal transudate, desquamated cells and secretions. When there is irritation or soreness, and

---

*See Findlay, *Reproduction and the Fetus*, Chapter 3

when the discharge is purulent, blood stained, offensive or profuse something is wrong and investigation is essential. Discharge is sometimes used as an introduction to the doctor when, in reality, there is another problem, e.g. sexual or marital difficulty.

Dysmenorrhoea

A certain amount of pain with the period is normal, but it should not incapacitate or distress anyone. It may be colicky or aching and present in the lower abdomen, radiate down the thighs or affect the back. Some bowel disturbance is not uncommon. The use of mild analgesics is sensible, and there is no reason to discourage women who feel they need relief from taking them. If mild analgesics are inadequate specialist advice is well justified.

Premenstrual tension is common in mild degree but if it interferes with work, causes family stress or misery to the sufferer, then it is not mild, not acceptable and help is needed by the patient. Doctors are not always as sympathetic as they might be towards compaints such as dysmenorrhoea and premenstrual tension, although it is essential in each case to find out how the problem affects the patient and why she is motivated to seek advice.

There is similar confusion over sexual activity particularly as there are fewer people qualified to give advice. Pain on intercourse is abnormal though it often occurs without there being any causative pelvic pathology. Bleeding after intercourse (postcoital) is always abnormal. If the woman loses her interest in sex, does not respond to sexual stimulation or reach orgasm, her sexuality is less than full and she should be given help if she will accept it (see Chapter 20).

Puberty*

This is a period of endocrine activity and development which leads to reproductive and sexual maturity. The release of gonadotrophins by the anterior pituitary gland results in the production of oestrogens by the ovary and body fat. This combined with androgens from the adrenal cortex and the ovary produce the characteristic changes of puberty: breast development (thelarche), the growth of axillary and pubic hair (adrenarche), development of the internal and external genitalia, deposition of fat around hips and buttocks, the growth spurt, and the first menstruation (menarche). This is a period of change for the girl and it is important that she be prepared for her emotional and physical development. Puberty may occur early (precocious), this is due, occasionally, to a tumour of the ovary or adrenal cortex.°

Menarche

This is defined as the age at which the first period occurs. The average age is 13 but the range of normal extends from 11–15. During the first year or two of menstruation the cycles may be anovular. These early periods are therefore

*See Findlay, *Reproduction and the Fetus*, Chapter 1
°For hormone levels during the stages of puberty see Findlay, *Reproduction and the Fetus*, Table 10.1.

often painless but may be heavy or irregular. Menorrhagia, dysmenorrhoea, amenorrhoea and failure of development may be problems during adolescence.

The climacteric

This is a period around the menopause (the 'last period') during which reproductive activity ceases. The menopause may come abruptly or there may be a gradual cessation of periods, anovular cycles, or irregular periods. During this time the disordered production of ovarian hormones may cause abnormal cycles, menorrhagia or symptoms of oestrogen deficiency (dyspareunia due to dryness of the vagina and hot flushes). Symptoms of oestrogen deficiency will normally respond to oestrogen; this is best given cyclically with additional progestogen during the second half of the cycle to avoid endometrial hyperplasia and the risk of endometrial carcinoma (see p 218.). Acceptance of the loss of fertility and reproductive function is not always easy, particularly if it is accompanied by distressing symptoms. Furthermore, it often coincides with the time when children are growing up or leave home and marital, social or occupational stresses may be great. Abnormal or irregular bleeding must not be attributed exclusively to the climacteric unless uterine or ovarian pathology has been excluded.

The menopause

Normally occurs between 45 and 52 years of age, with an average of 50. By definition, bleeding which occurs longer than 6 months after the apparent last period in women of this age group is classified as 'post menopausal' and must be investigated. After the menopause symptoms of oestrogen deficiency, as above, may require treatment. Physical changes will also occur, such as the redistribution of fat and breast atrophy. Bone loss may be accelerated after the menopause years but fractures due to osteoporosis generally occur a decade or two later.

Screening

The value of examining or investigating apparently healthy people for early or asymptomatic disease is controversial. Early diagnosis or prevention is an attractive proposition, but it is difficult to assess its value and cost-effectiveness. In our specialty family planning, antenatal and postnatal clinics are effectively screening clinics where medical disorders such as hypertension may be diagnosed for the first time, and where examination of the breasts, pelvic examination and cervical cytology is used to exclude disease as far as possible (Table 14.1). Self-referral to specialist clinics (for sexually transmitted disease) and family planning clinics, gives women access to screening and expert advice. Doctors do not have to do all the screening, since trained nurses can examine breasts, take smears and carry out pelvic examinations.

Some women practice self-examination of the breasts and this is to be encouraged. It takes only a few moments to examine the breasts of a woman attending a gynaecological clinic; many gynaecologists do this and many women appreciate it. Cervical smears can also be taken as part of a pelvic examination with minimal effort. The processing and reporting of the smear requires finance, but if the patient goes to a doctor for a smear, the doctor will be paid to take it. Similarly the provision of mammography for screening large numbers of women has to be justified in terms of absence of harmful effects, reduced morbidity and mortality and effective use of financial investment. We need to know whether diagnosing and treating early carcinoma and cervical intraepithelial neoplasia (CIN) can prevent the development of invasive carcinoma and lead to a reduced mortality rate from this disease. The evidence so far is that early diagnosis and treatment after cytology will markedly reduce the rate of invasive carcinoma of the cervix.

Table 14.1 Deaths in 1980 and 1981 from carcinoma of the breast, ovary and cervix (England and Wales).

	1980	1981
Carcinoma of the breast	12167	12513
Carcinoma of the ovary (Includes other rare adnexal tumours)	3711	3709
Carcinoma of the cervix	2068	2017

In the UK general practitioners were only encouraged recently to take cervical smears from women over 35 and from younger women with more than 3 pregnancies, with repeat smears at 5 year intervals. Many gynaecologists take cervical smears in antenatal, family planning and gynaecological clinics. In North America the gynaecologists advocate annual smears, but the health authorities advise 3-yearly smears. The arguments are complicated by the risk of a false negative smear (due to an unrepresentative cell sample or misinterpretation) and the use of statistics, which indicate that most carcinomas of the cervix develop at 40–50 and the preinvasive stages last 10 years or more. These do not take account, however, of the increasing amount of invasive and preinvasive disease among younger women, even in their 20s.

At present it seems sensible for cervical smears to be taken from women who are, or have been sexually active, starting in the early twenties (cervical carcinoma is very rare in virgins). Those who attend antenatal, family planning, sexually transmitted disease and gynaecological clinics should have smears taken at intervals of perhaps three years or when they attend. Others should have at least two smears before 30 and regular smears at 3–5 yearly intervals thereafter until 60–70.

Further reading

Brook C.G.D. (1981). Delayed puberty. *British Journal of Hospital Medicine* **26**,6,573–580.
Chamberlain, J. (1982). Screening for cancer. *Hospital Medicine* **276**, 583–591.

Draper, G.J. and Cook G.A. (1983). Changing patterns of cervical cancer rates. *British Medical Journal* 287, 511–5.

Wolfendale, M.R., King S. and Usherwood, M.McD. (1983). Abnormal cervical smears; are we in for an epidemic? *British Medical Journal* **287**, 526–528.

15

Family planning

Family planning implies that couples should be able to have children when they wish to do so and to use effective contraceptive measures when they do not. Therefore, doctors should be able to give advice about contraception and to help when couples have difficulty with conception (infertility or subfertility). The ethical background to this concept is often left unmentioned in undergraduate textbooks; the decisions about such matters being the responsibility and choice of the individual.

Professionals and laypeople often seem unaware of the problems of overpopulation; the poverty of many families, and the deprivation, neglect and cruelty to which children can be subjected. While policies on population, living standards and finance for health and family planning services are political decisions, the medical profession is greatly involved in such issues both at a national level and with individual patients.

The aim that every child should be a wanted child is still far from realization; the need for therapeutic abortion, adoption and the fate of unwanted children emphasize how far we have to go. In particular the education of the young about sex, marriage and parenthood is still inadequate; they need to be encouraged to reflect on some of the implications of parenthood, the satisfaction of having a child, the companionship and the pride in its achievements on one hand; but the anxiety, loss of privacy, lowered standard of living and additional work on the other. Any contribution in this area by doctors advising men and women, must include appreciation of the social situation, the problems and ethical viewpoint of the individual couple, and an involvement in health education.

Contraception

All methods are liable to failure and have potential disadvantages so that choice is often not easy. The methods can be grouped as follows:

1. Barrier.
2. Hormonally induced contraception.
3. Intrauterine devices (IUCDs).
4. Coitus interruptus.
5. Safe period (rhythm).

6. Post coital contraception.

7. Sterilization.

It should be remembered that it is the woman who almost always has most to lose from failure, and whose motivation towards contraception is strongest, so that methods under her control may be preferable. Ideally, however, the choice of method should be a joint decision by a couple, subject to the relationship being marital or stable; this is well illustrated by the choice of sterilization when either partner can undergo the operation.

Barrier methods

These methods should always be used with a spermicide such as Nonoxynol which may be delivered as a cream, gel, pessary or foam. A spermicide or barrier on its own is not reliable enough. Occasionally there is allergy to spermicide or to rubber.

The Sheath (condom, 'French Letter')

This is worn on the penis and collects the ejaculate. Spill may occur, and lead to pregnancy, if the penis is not withdrawn before loss of an erection. It should preferably be used with a spermicide because of the risk of spill or bursting. It has the advantage of not requiring medical advice or prescription and affords some protection against sexually transmitted disease.

The diaphragm

This is a rubber device fitted so that it is held above the pubic bone anteriorly and in the posterior vaginal fornix posteriorly covering the cervix, (Fig. 15.1).

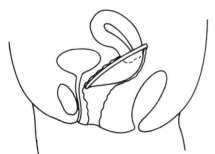

Fig. 15.1   Vaginal diaphragm.

The device must be fitted by a doctor and inserted by the patient and should be refitted every 6 months and after pregnancy. It must be comfortable and the woman should be unaware of it. Jelly or cream is usually applied to both surfaces of the diaphragm which must be left in place 6–8 hours after the last intercourse. If intercourse occurs, or is repeated more than 3 hours after insertion a further application of spermicide is required (using an applicator to save removing and replacing the diaphragm). It is occasionally unsuitable because of uterine or vaginal prolapse and some women find it inconvenient and messy to use. It is an efficient method with few side effects (allergy to rubber or spermicide is the commonest) if it is used conscientiously after proper fitting, instruction and practice in its use. The failure rate can be as low as 2–3 per 100 woman years, similar to that for the IUCD.

Cervical caps, vault caps and vimules are other mechanical barriers occasionally used. The vault cap adheres by suction and the cervical cap and vimule fit over the cervix.

Hormonal contraception

Oestrogen-Progestogen combined contraceptive pills

These generally suppress ovulation by acting at the hypothalamic-pituitary level. They also affect the endometrium, the cervical mucus and the mechanics of ovum transport, so that if ovulation does occur there are other 'back up' contraceptive actions.

The pills are normally packed for 21 day courses and are taken from the first day of the cycle. A withdrawal bleed should follow 2 days after the last tablet but in any event they should be restarted after seven days or ovulation and pregnancy may occur. If 'the pill' is started after the first day of the cycle the patient is at risk of pregnancy in that cycle and must take other precautions for fourteen days from when she takes the first pill.

Choice of pill
A list of combined pills is given in Table 15.1, divided according to progestogen. The guiding principle is to select a low dose pill, i.e. one containing less than 50μg of oestrogen and a low dose of progestogen, and to change to a stronger pill if necessary. For example low doses of progestogen are more frequently associated with break through bleeding. ED (Every Day) preparations are useful for those who are forgetful; when starting, the first pill is taken from the appropriate 'blister' section of the pack on the first day of bleeding, but extra contraceptive precautions are required for 14 days. (These packs contain 28 pills, 7 of which are dummies).

Changing Preparations
No additional precautions are required if changing to a higher dose pill. If changing to a lower dose pill, start the new brand without any gap after stopping the old one.

The combined contraceptive pill has a very low failure rate of 0.1 per 100 woman years. It gives a regular predictable cycle usually free of dysmenorrhoea and premenstrual tension with reduced menstrual loss. For these reasons and because of the simplicity of taking a pill regularly it is welcomed by many women. A disadvantage, however, is the need for medical supervision because of the serious complications which occasionally occur (see below), the need to prescribe an appropriate pill for each individual and the problems which may occur in relation to its use.

Table 15.1 Combined contraceptive pills used in the UK and their American equivalent

Name	Manufacturer	Progestogen mg	Oestrogen μg	Pills/pack	American equivalent
Norinyl–1	Syntex	Norethisterone 1.0	Mestranol 50	21	Norinyl 1/50
Norinyl 28	Syntex	Norethisterone 1.0	Mestranol 50	21 + 7 blank	Norinyl 28
Ortho–Novin 1/50	Ortho–Cilag	Norethisterone 1.0	Mestranol 50	21	Ortho–novum
—	Mead Johnson	Norethisterone 1.0	Mestranol 50	21	Ovcon 50
Norimin	Syntex	Norethisterone 1.0	Ethinyloestradiol 35	21	Norinyl 1/35
Ovysmen	Ortho–Cilag	Norethisterone 0.5	Ethinyloestradiol 35	21	Modicon
Brevinor	Syntex	Norethisterone 0.5	Ethinyloestradiol 35	21	Brevicon
—	Mead Johnson	Norethisterone 0.4	Ethinyloestradiol 35	21	Ovcon 35
—	Parke–Davis	Norethisterone 1.5	Ethinyloestradiol 30	21	Loestrin 1.5/30
Anovlar	Schering	Norethisterone acetate 4.0	Ethinyloestradiol 50	21	—
Gynovlar	Schering	Norethisterone acetate 3.0	Ethinyloestradiol 50	21	—
Norlestrin	Parke–Davis	Norethisterone acetate 2.5	Ethinyloestradiol 50	21	Norlestrin 2.5/50
Minovlar	Schering	Norethisterone acetate 1.0	Ethinyloestradiol 50	21	Norlestrin 1/50 (Parke–Davis)*
Minovlar ED	Schering	Norethisterone acetate 1.0	Ethinyloestradiol 50	21 + 7 blank	—
Orlest 21	Parke–Davis	Norethisterone acetate 1.0	Ethinyloestradiol 50	21	Norlestrin 1/50
Loestrin	Parke–Davis	Norethisterone acetate 1.0	Ethinyloestradiol 20	21	Loestrin 1/20
Ovulen 50	Gold Cross	Ethynodiol diacetate 1.0	Ethinyloestradiol 50	21	Demulen†
Conova 30	Gold Cross	Ethynodiol diacetate 2.0	Ethinyloestradiol 50	21	—
Minilyn	Organon	Lynestrenol 2.5	Ethinyloestradiol 50	22	—
Ovran	Wyeth	Levonorgestrel 0.25	Ethinyloestradiol 50	21	—
—	Wyeth	Levonorgestrel 0.5	Ethinyloestradiol 50	21	Ovral
Eugynon 50	Schering	Levonorgestrel 0.25	Ethinyloestradiol 50	21	—
Ovran 30	Wyeth	Levonorgestrel 0.25	Ethinyloestradiol 30	21	—
Eugynon 30	Schering	Levonorgestrel 0.25	Ethinyloestradiol 30	21	—
Ovranette	Wyeth	Levonorgestrel 0.15	Ethinyloestradiol 30	21	Nordette
Microgynon 30	Schering	Levonorgestrel 0.15	Ethinyloestradiol 30	21	—
—	Wyeth	Levonorgestrel 0.3	Ethinyloestradiol 30	21	Looval 0.5

Name	Manufacturer	Progestogen mg	Oestrogen μg	Pills/pack	American equivalent
Marvelon	Organon	Desogestrel 0.15	Ethinyloestradiol 30	21	—
Biphasic					
Binovum	Ortho–Cilag	Norethisterone 0.5	Ethinyloestradiol 35	7	—
		Norethisterone 1.0	Ethinyloestradiol 35	14	—
—	Ortho–Cilag	Norethisterone 0.5	Ethinyloestradiol 35	10	Orthonovum
		Norethisterone 1.0	Ethinyloestradiol 35	10	
Triphasic					
Logynon	Schering	Levonorgestrel 0.05	Ethinyloestradiol 30	6	—
		Levonorgestrel 0.075	Ethinyloestradiol 40	5	
		Levonorgestrel 0.125	Ethinyloestradiol 30	10	
Logynon ED	Schering	Levonorgestrel 0.05	Ethinyloestradiol 30	6	—
		Levonorgestrel 0.075	Ethinyloestradiol 40	5 + 7 blank	
		Levonorgestrel 0.125	Ethinyloestradiol 30	10	
Trinordiol	Wyeth	Levonorgestrel 0.05	Ethinyloestradiol 30	6	—
		Levonorgestrel 0.075	Ethinyloestradiol 40	5	
		Levonorgestrel 0.125	Ethinyloestradiol 30	11	
Trinovum	Ortho–Cilag	Norethisterone 0.5	Ethinyloestradiol 35	7	—
		Norethisterone 0.75	Ethinyloestradiol 35	7	
		Norethisterone 1.0	Ethinyloestradiol 35	7	

Note, see Appendix II for the American names of the progestogens and oestrogens used.
*The equivalent pill by a different manufacturer.
†Do not confuse this with Demulen 1/35; Ethynodiol 1.0 mg. Ethinyloestradiol 35 μg.

Health aspects of the pill

The pill reduces the incidence of physiological ovarian cysts, benign breast disease and pelvic inflammatory disease. The first recognised danger was thromboembolic disease; later myocardial infarction, cerebrovascular accidents, arterial thrombosis, hypertension and hepatic adenoma were identified as rare but serious complications. The oestrogen appears to be responsible for most of the complications, but the progestogen or its ratio to oestrogen is responsible for reducing high density lipoprotein cholesterol (HDL-cholesterol); a high level of which appears to protect against atheroma. Oestrogen and progestogen affect carbohydrate metabolism adversely.

Recent papers, as yet uncorroborated, suggest that some pills taken for at least five years may increase the risk of breast carcinoma, while another defines a possible link between very long term use of combined pills and carcinoma of the cervix. Media reports of papers of this type cause great alarm and are rarely objective. Such events emphasize the need for women to make an informed decision about taking the pill; this requires consideration of the risks and benefits, not only of the pill, but also of other usually less reliable alternative methods of contraception. It also adds impetus to the preference for low dose pills.

Before prescribing the pill

Take a careful history and examine the patient to exclude high risk factors:

1. Age — the pill is generally contraindicated after 45.
2. Cigarette smoking — the pill is generally contraindicated after 35 because of the increased risk of coronary artery disease.
3. Abnormal plasma lipids — clue from history of circulatory disease in young relatives; high cholesterol is an absolute contraindication.
4. Previous vascular disease — thrombosis, embolism are absolute contraindications.
5. Diabetes.
6. Obesity.
7. Hypertension.
8. Disease which may be adversely affected by the pill e.g. carcinoma of the breast, active liver disease, diabetes mellitus.

Acquaint the patient with the risk in relative terms, your advice and the alternatives available. Remember to balance the risk of oral contraceptives with those of pregnancy, everyday life and the woman's preferences. If prescribing the pill, use a low dose preparation (see Table 15.1) and watch for the development of risk factors (e.g. hypertension).

Beneficial side effects

1 .Menstruation regular, reduced loss, premenstrual tension and dysmenorrhoea.
2 .Less benign breast disease, ovarian cyst formation, pelvic inflammatory disease.
3 .May reduce effects of fibroids, endometriosis.

Adverse side effects
1. No withdrawal bleed, breakthrough bleeding, cervical erosion.
2. Headache, migraine (usually while off the pill), fluid retention, weight gain.
3. Nausea and breast tenderness are quite common on starting the pill.

Rare side effects
1. The serious side effects include gallstones, coronary thrombosis, hypertension, jaundice, venous or arterial thrombosis, embolism.
2. Less serious but significant side effects include chloasma (pigmentation of the face as in pregnancy), and dyspareunia (due to dryness).
3. Depression and loss of libido are frequently attributed to the pill, but the relationship is not proven.

The missed pill
If a pill is missed but the patient remembers within 12 hours and therefore takes it within 36 hours she can continue regular pill taking without extra precautions.

If more than one pill has been missed, or longer than 36 hours have elapsed since the last pill, the omitted pill/pills should be taken as soon as possible, followed by others in the normal way. There is a risk of pregnancy and another contraceptive method should be used for 14 days. If there is any suggestion of pregnancy or no withdrawal bleed, medical advice should be sought.

Other causes of failure
Diarrhoea and vomiting may prevent absorption of the pill and other precautions or another pill must be taken after vomiting. In addition certain drugs act as enzyme inducers and accclerate metabolism so that low dose pills may be inadequate. These include rifampicin, phenobarbitone, phenytoin, primidone, griseofulvin, carbamazepine and dichloralphenazone. Antibiotics such as ampicillin and tetracycline may cause diarrhoea and affect absorption.

Fertility after the pill
There is no long-term impairment, but it seems that women coming off the pill may take up to three months longer to conceive than those discontinuing other methods. This is, in part, due to the delay which may occur before ovulation occurs, often appreciably longer than two weeks. Amenorrhoea affects about 1 per cent of women stopping the pill and should be investigated in the normal way (see p. 166).

The pill after pregnancy
After a termination or spontaneous abortion the pill may be started the next day. For women breast-feeding the combined pill is generally regarded as best avoided (see p. 153 — progestogen-only-pill). For those not breast-feeding it should be started three weeks after delivery without waiting for a period, or use an alternative method until the first period after which the pill can be taken in the normal way.

Progestogen only pills (POP)

These are listed in Table 15.2. These are taken daily without any break, they do not suppress ovulation in most women and act by their effect on the cervical mucus and endometrium. It is vital to take this pill at the same time each day (the early evening is ideal since there is then maximal protection around bedtime). It is started on the first day of a period and additional measures are required for 14 days. If the woman vomits within 2 hours of taking the pill, or has diarrhoea 12 to 24 hours later, she should use an additional method for 14 days. The failure rate is between 1 and 4 pregnancies per 100 woman years with an increased risk of ectopic pregnancy. Because it does not appear to affect coagulation it is useful for older women, smokers, diabetics and some with hypertension. It is contraindicated after ectopic pregnancy but can be taken while breast-feeding.

Table 15.2 Progestogen only pills.

	Progestogen	Dose µg	Pill/pack
Femulen (Gold Cross)	Ethynodiol diacetate	500	28
Micronor (Ortho–Cilag)	Norethisterone	350	28
Microval (Wyeth)	Levonorgestrel	30	35
Neogest (Schering)	Norgestrel	75	35
Norgeston (Schering)	Levonorgestrel	30	35
Noriday (Syntex)	Norethisterone	350	28

Depot injections of medroxyprogesterone acetate 150–300 mg

Intramuscular injection either during the first 5 days of the cycle or after delivery (optimally in the first week but later if necessary). Irregular bleeding, spotting or erratic periods may occur in 25 per cent of women. There has been some political opposition to its use on the grounds of lack of informed consent; it is generally wise to restrict it to women who are being immunized against rubella and those whose husbands have undergone vasectomy and are awaiting clearance (see p. 156). One dose may last 3 months with a failure rate comparable to that of the combined pill. It seems to have a beneficial effect in reducing the frequency of sickle cell crises.

Intrauterine devices (IUCDs)

These are made of plastic, sometimes with added copper. Examples are shown in Fig. 15.2 and new designs appear regularly. These devices once inserted should provide contraception until they are removed. The copper devices are normally changed after two to three years but the Novagard is now permitted to be used for 4 years. One device incorporates progesterone and this lasts one year only. It reduces the menstrual loss in contrast to most devices but is not widely used. A newer version incorporating levonorgestrel may be used longer.

Insertion is painful sometimes, particularly for nulliparous patients;

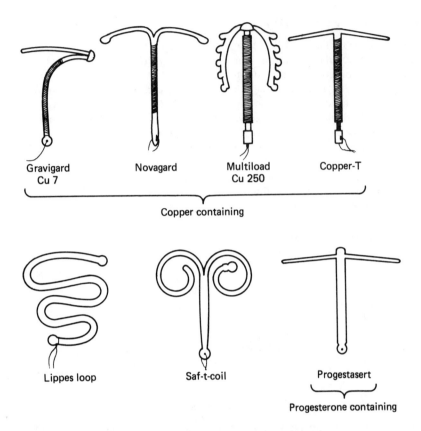

Fig. 15.2 Intrauterine contraceptive devices (IUCDs) currently in use.

there appears to be an increased risk of pelvic inflammatory disease in young nulliparous women. At least part of their action appears to involve the prevention of implantation; removal before the latter half of the cycle may therefore be followed by pregnancy, so is best avoided unless other contraceptive measures are taken for a week prior to removal or contraception is not required.

Contraindications
These devices should not be given to women who may be pregnant, who may have active or recent pelvic inflammatory or sexually transmitted disease, previous ectopic pregnancy, an abnormal uterus, abnormal uterine bleeding or immunosuppression.

Caution should be exercised with the young, especially those with previous pelvic inflammation, diabetes mellitus (risk of infection), cardiovascular disease (there is an increased risk of endocarditis), endometriosis, severe dysmenorrhoea and menorrhagia.

In general these devices seem best suited for older women (failure rate 0.5 per 100 women years over 35). Complications include syncope at insertion, perforation of the uterus, pain, pelvic infection and abnormal bleeding. The amount and duration of menstrual loss is normally increased by a device. Expulsion may occur and the patient is usually checked 6 weeks after insertion and then 6-monthly, while she herself can check its presence by feeling for the nylon thread. If this is not felt she should contact the doctor and use alternative contraception (if it has come out however, she may already be pregnant). On examination the device can often be located in the uterus by a sound (easiest at period time), vabra curette or a specially designed instrument, provided the patient is not pregnant. Ultrasound or X-rays may be helpful if it is not found by other methods, particularly if it has perforated the uterus.

Should pregnancy occur in spite of a device in the uterus there is an increased risk of ectopic pregnancy (which must be excluded) and of abortion in the first and second trimesters. It is often possible to remove devices in the early weeks without disturbing the pregnancy, this is advisable in order to reduce the risk of abortion and infection.

Coitus interruptus

This involves withdrawal of the penis just before ejaculation, failure may occur either because withdrawal is too late or there is spillage of sperm in the vagina or on the vulva. It is a traditional method but unreliable and disturbs the climax of coitus. In spite of this withdrawal is widely used and acceptable to many couples for whom it greatly reduces the risk of pregnancy.

The safe period

This does not actually exist. The method ('rhythm') is based on avoiding days immediately before and after ovulation but ovulation is never entirely predictable, cycles vary, and there is limited survival of ovum (perhaps 1–2 days) and spermatozoa (up to 4 days). For a 28 day cycle abstinence was traditionally recommended from day 10–16, but reliability is improved if abstinence is extended to cover the pattern of previous cycle variability or a temperature chart or mucus observation used. Coitus after ovulation is safer than before and the longer the period of abstinence the more reliable the method.

Postcoital contraception

A high protection rate can be achieved either by inserting an intrauterine device within 5 days of the coitus or by taking a pill (containing 250µg levonorgestrel and 50µg ethinyloestradiol) in a dose of 2 tablets, repeated after exactly 12 hours, not longer than 72 hours after intercourse. The patients must be aware of the implications if the method fails and follow up is essential. This is a method for emergency use only and it requires medical supervision.

Sterlization

This is a permanent and generally reliable method of contraception. Though reversal and subsequent pregnancy is sometimes possible, it should be regarded as irreversible for counselling purposes. It is best if couples can discuss it with more than one person so that they are fully aware of all the implications and have ample time to reconsider their decision before the operation is performed. Important points include.

1. The exact surgical procedure.
2. The effects of sterilization (generally minimal to the healthy well-adjusted person).
3. The possibility of loss of children or remarriage.
4. The risk of failure, which must be understood and accepted.
5. If appropriate, the effect of coming off the pill or having an IUCD out (respectively heavier or lighter periods).

Younger people, those with unstable marriages and those who have sterilizations with termination of pregnancy, or soon after delivery (which are bad times for decision making), are statistically most likely to regret the decision.

Vasectomy is an outpatient procedure for most men, but the man cannot

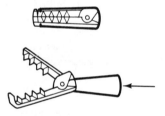

Fig. 15.3 Samaritan clip based on the Hulka-Clemens clip.

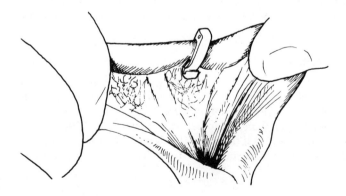

Fig. 15.4 Filshie clip applied to a tube.

rely on it until he has had 2 negative semen counts, often 12 weeks later. Sterilization of the woman generally involves a brief admission to hospital, varying from one or 2–7 nights. Many surgeons use the laparoscope to apply clips or rings, (Fig. 15.3), alternatively the tubes can be clipped, destroyed with diathermy, divided or excised through a small or 'mini-laparotomy', or occasionally by the vaginal route.

Termination of pregnancy

The availability of abortion for unwanted early pregnancies depends on the law of the country, the attitude of the population and doctors, and access to those who can provide it. Prevention of unwanted pregnancy by contraception must always be preferable to abortion, but it is difficult to imagine a world in which there will not be unwanted pregnancies due to failure to use contraception, misuse or method failures. For patients who have moral objections to termination it is not an option. Professional staff are entitled to choose whether or not to be involved in counselling or operations for termination.

Where abortion is permitted by law there are usually situations or conditions specified, as in the 1967 Abortion Act in the United Kingdom:

1. The continuance of the pregnancy would involve risk to the life of the pregnant woman greater than if the pregnancy were terminated.
2. The continuance of the pregnancy would involve risk to the physical or mental health of the pregnant woman greater than if the pregnancy were terminated.
3. The continuance of the pregnancy would involve risk of injury to the physical or mental health of the existing children of the family of the pregnant woman greater than if the pregnancy were terminated.
4. There is substantial risk that if the child were born it would suffer from such physical or mental abnormalities as to be seriously handicapped.

Counselling

This is the essential preliminary to abortion. It involves discussion with the woman and preferably her partner as well. This may be done by doctors alone, or with the help of social workers or others according to the situation and will include.

1. The reason for seeking abortion.
2. Any reason for advising abortion (maternal ill-health, risk of fetal abnormalities etc.).
3. Discussion of relevant factors; marital status or prospects, family, housing , career, finance, etc.
4. The method and implications of termination.
5. Implications for future pregnancy.
6. The risk of complications and their nature.
7. The prevention of further unwanted pregnancy.
8. What does the woman herself really want?

Two doctors must certify the need and reasons for termination.

Methods of termination

In the first trimester abortion is best accomplished by suction curettage under local or general anaesthesia. The risks include incomplete abortion (see p. 94) incompetence of the cevix if this is overdilated, and pelvic infection.

Second trimester abortion is more dangerous and also more distressing for patient and staff due to the methods involved and the more advanced stage of the pregnancy. Many methods have been and still are used including hysterotomy (like early caesarean section) and intra-amniotic injection of prostaglandin and urea; perhaps the preferable method at present is the extra-amniotic injection of prostaglandin E_2 through a catheter introduced into the cervix (see Appendix for dosage and side effects).

Emotional support and analgesics will be required during the abortion and the stress for the patient varies greatly, particularly depending on her emotional state and the reason for termination.

Incomplete abortion, haemorrhage and sepsis are possible complications, and the uterus should be explored if the abortion is incomplete.

Infertility

Approximately 10 per cent of couples fail to achieve a pregnancy at all, while more than 70 per cent of couples succeed within 12 months. It is, therefore, appropriate for couples to seek advice after a year. In some cases they may be justified in going to the doctor earlier if they know or suspect something is wrong. Often there is pressure from relatives or marital stress; almost always there is considerable anxiety which may increase under the pressure of investigation or treatment. It is the doctor's responsibility to provide support and reassurance for the couple, to give an honest assessment of the chances of conception and to regulate any investigation or treatment so that too much pressure is not put upon the couple. Some who come to infertility clinics do conceive but have suffered abortion or obstetric disasters and seek an explanation of their past misfortune and treatment or reassurance for the future. Others have a history of disease or require genetic counselling. Sexual problems are common among infertile couples and can also be created or aggravated by investigation and treatment. The best way to start the investigation of infertility is to see the husband and wife separately, take a history from, and examine each partner and then discuss the situation, possible investigations and treatment with the couple together.

Factors contributing to or causing infertility may be classified as follows:

1. The semen e.g. azoospermia, oligospermia or poor motility.
2. The mucus and cervix — e.g. inadequate mucus.
3. The uterus — e.g. submucous fibroid, congenital abnormality.
4. Tubal damage — e.g. obstruction from pelvic inflammatory disease.
5. Peritoneal changes — e.g. adhesions from pelvic inflammatory disease.
6. Ovulation — e.g. anovulation or irregular ovulation, short luteal phase.
7. Sexual — e.g. apareunia, dyspareunia, ejaculatory dysfunction.
8. Religion, by custom may interfere with sexual activity or investigation — e.g. the Jewish restriction on coitus after menstruation.

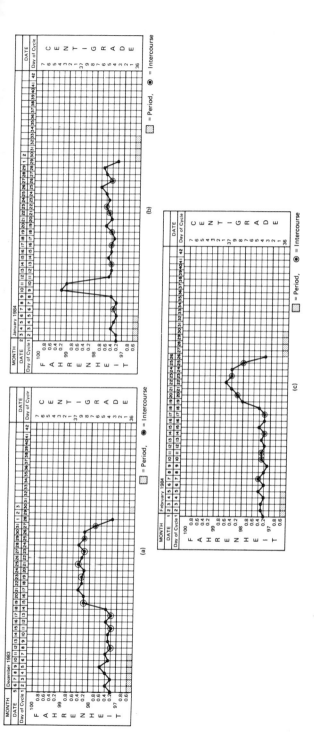

Fig. 15.5   Women's temperature charts showing (a) ovulatory cycle, (b) anovulatory cycle and (c) short luteal phase.

9. Social; living conditions, occupation and family relationships may be relevant — partners separated while one works away from home, lack of privacy at home or night work reducing the frequency of intercourse;
10. Medical; general disease — e.g. diabetes mellitus. Cytotoxic drugs may produce temporary or permanent azoospermia. Salazopyrin, androgens and anabolic steroids can cause oligospermia while the hypotensive agents and phenothiazines may cause impotence.

Some couples seek advice but do not necessarily wish to have a child immediately; others such as alcoholics, battered wives and those with unstable marriages, may be better helped to solve their other problems before having children.

Investigations which may be helpful include:

Semen test

The sample obtained by masturbation should have;
1. volume of 1.5–5 ml.
2. a concentration of more than 20×10^6 spermatozoa/ml, not more than 25 per cent abnormal forms
3. more than 30 per cent spermatozoa showing progressive motility.

If the test is below normal it should be repeated since there can be wide variations. Recent illness may have an adverse effect, spermatogenesis takes about 11 weeks and an appropriate interval should therefore elapse before the test is repeated.

The temperature chart

The woman takes her temperature before she gets up in the morning. The chart gives a reasonably accurate indication whether ovulation is occurring as well as a record of cycles and information about timing and frequency of coitus. It is not a very accurate way of timing ovulation and patients should not time coitus strictly from the chart for this reason (see Fig. 15.5).

Postcoital Test

A sample of mucus is aspirated from the cervical canal within 16 hours of intercourse during the preovulatory phase. The mucus is judged by its quantity, viscosity, spinnbarkeit (ability to be drawn out in a thread), and the presence of spermatozoa which should show progressive motility in the mucus. Leucocytes and bacteria suggest infection which should be further investigated.

Unsatisfactory tests may be due to inadequate oestrogen, poor semen, faulty sexual technique or antisperm antibodies. Crossmatch testing (using donor semen and mucus), antibody tests (e.g. the Isojima) and microbiological investivation of both partners may be helpful.

Hysterosalpingography

A radio-opaque substance is injected into the cervix to outline the uterine

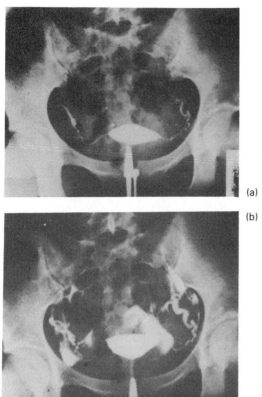

(a)

(b)

Fig.15.6 Hysterosalpingography:
(a) filling of the uterus and tubes,
(b) intraperitoneal spill of dye.

cavity and tubes. It should pass into the peritoneal cavity freely (Fig. 15.6).
This is a good means of detecting submucous fibroids, congenital
abnormalities, and tubal blockage. If done without ananaesthetic it can be
painful and there is a risk of infection (probably about 1 per cent). It does not
show peritoneal adhesions or the ovaries and some gynaecologists therefore
prefer laparoscopy.

Laparoscopy

This enable the uterus, tubes and ovaries to be inspected. Evidence of
ovulation may be seen and the patency of the tubes can be checked by
injecting dye through the cervix. This is usually done under general
anaesthesia, and therefore involves the risks of laparoscopy and anaesthesia.

Endometrial biopsy or curettage

The cavity of the uterus can be checked with forceps and a curette for polyps, congenital abnormalities and fibroids; tissue obtained in this way can be sent for histological and/or microbiological examination. The histology should fit with the stage of the cycle. Culture is necessary for the diagnosis of tuberculosis for which the biopsy should be taken immediately premenstrually.

Serum progesterone

This is an indirect means of confirming ovulation. The level should be greater than 25 nmol/litre 5–8 days before the start of a period.

Other useful investigations

Hysteroscopy, chromosome studies (for those with recurrent abortion and men with possible Klinefelter's syndrome), and measurements of gonadotrophins and sex steroids in women with suspected ovarian failure or polycystic ovarian disease, or in men with azoospermia. Testicular biopsy may occasionally be justifed if the vas deferens is thought to be occluded, but this procedure can cause antibody formation. Ultrasound may be used to identify ovarian activity, folicular ripening and rupture, ovarian polycystic conditions and uterine fibroids (Fig. 15.7). For the investigations of amenorrhoea see p. 166.

Treatment

Simple measures, such as changing from tight supportive (jockey) underpants to the looser (boxer) type may produce a significant improvement in sperm count or motility. In appropriate cases reduction of weight, alcohol intake and smoking may be effective. Ligation of a varicocele may be justified to reduce the temperature within the scrotum. Androgens are not useful but gonadotrophin or GnRH (releasing hormone) therapy, or vasal surgery (for occlusion) may be justified occasionally.

Failure to ovulate, or to do so regularly, may be treated with clomiphene, tamoxifen, cyclofenyl, gonadotrophin or GnRH (see Appendix). It is difficult to investigate patients who are not ovulating or have long or irregular cycles. It is therefore often wise to induce regular ovulation; this may be followed by pregnancy and if not further investigation is easier.

If the postcoital test is unsatisfactory, the quality of the cervical mucus may be improved by small doses of an oestrogen (e.g. 10µg ethinyloestradiol for 3–4 days before ovulation). Precoital alkaline douching is often advised but its value is not clear. The value of Artificial Insemination by Husband (AIH) is difficult to assess except when normal coitus cannot, or does not occur.

Tubal blockage or intraperitoneal adhesion may be treated by surgery, but before undertaking this it is important for patient and doctor to accept that there is no guarantee of success. Both tubal surgery and pelvic inflammation alike predispose to ectopic pregnancy, and pelvic inflammatory disease is liable to recur.

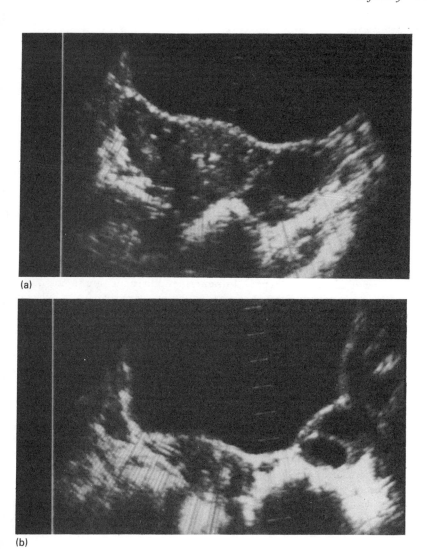

(a)

(b)

Fig. 15.7   Ultrasound showing; (a) one ripe ovarian follicle and (b) two ovarian follicles.

The operations can be categorized as follows:

Salpingolysis
Division of adhesions which cover or distort the tube or block the fimbrial end.

Salpingostomy
Surgical opening of a tube blocked at the fimbrial end, the fimbria may be reasonably well preserved or almost totally destroyed. The tube is normally stitched open.

Tubal anastomosis
Where the tube is blocked the obstructed portion may be removed and the tube anastomosed, in some cases over a splint. This operation is the normal means of reversing sterilization.

Tubal implant
If the interstitial portion of the tube is blocked and the remainder of the tube patent, the cornu of the uterus may be opened and the patent tube introduced and sutured in place.

Oolysis
Adhesions over the ovaries may be removed. Some surgeons use microsurgery as the tube is so narrow, particularly medially. The best results are obtained with simple operations and when there has been little tubal damage; as with oolysis, salpingolysis and reversal of sterilization where pregnancy rates of 50 per cent are attainable.

Surgery is also appropriate for submucous fibroids and occasionally to excise congenital uterine septa. Intrauterine adhesions are seen quite frequently in some countries and can be treated by surgery and prophylactic insertion of an intrauterine device.

With women over 40 the justifiable extent of investigation and treatment is particularly difficult to define. In discussion with patients the realistic chance of achieving success, the implications of pregnancy at that age and the risks of investigation need to be explained carefully and balanced.

In up to 20 per cent of couples no explanation will be found for the infertility, pregnancy may occur in many of these couples though we have no way of predicting the chance for one couple. For those unlikely to succeed on the basis of the investigations described; adoption, artificial insemination by donor (AID) and *in vitro* fertilization (IVF) are possible solutions. Though these methods are not generally available and have ethical and other implications which are not acceptable to everyone.
For some the reassurance of investigations which are normal is helpful, for others the discovery that they are unlikely to have a child is sad, but the ending of uncertainty often comes as a relief.

Further reading

Guillebaud J. (1983). *The Pill*. Oxford University Press, Oxford.
Potts, M. and Diggory, P.L.C. (1983). *Textbook of Contraceptive Practice*. Cambridge University Press, Cambridge.
International Planned Parenthood Federation (1980). *Family Planning Handbook for Doctors*. IPPF, London.

16

Abnormal menstruation and vaginal bleeding

Primary amenorrhoea

Lack of menstruation is a symptom. As 95 per cent of adolescents will have menstruated by the age of 16, it is appropriate to investigate girls with amenorrhoea at this age and earlier if there is any reason to suspect that something is amiss. For example the genitalia seem abnormal or appearances suggest a syndrome, such as Turner's, associated with ovarian dysgenesis. Primary amenorrhoea is relatively uncommon and a detailed description of the differential diagnosis and investigation is beyond the scope of this book. A classification of causes is given in Table 16.1 but is not intended to be comprehensive. The history of the girl must include details of the physical development and any previous illness or treatment. Occasionally removal or destruction of the ovaries is revealed as the cause.

Table 16.1 Aetiology of primary amenorrhoea.

Central nervous system:	Disease of the hypothalamus
	Deficiency of gonadotrophin releasing hormone (GnRh)
	Polycystic ovarian disease
	Drugs, (phenothiazines, steroids)
	Psychogenic (Anorexia nervosa, stress)
Pituitary fossa:	Tumours (prolactinoma, acromegaly)
	Gonadotrophin deficiency syndromes
General disease:	Thyroid dysfunction
	Severe illness (diabetes, cirrhosis, nephritis, tuberculosis)
	Adrenal disorders (congenital adrenal hyperplasia)
	Nutritional (anorexia nervosa, weight loss, athletes and dancers).
Gonadal disorders:	Dysgenesis (e.g. Turner's Syndrome)
	Hermaphroditism (true hermaphroditism, androgen insensitivity)
	Ovarian failure (premature menopause)
	Destruction or removal
	Tumours (androgen producing, very rare)
Genital tract:	Vaginal membrane (cryptomenorrhoea)
	Absent vagina
	Absence of uterus
	Pelvic tuberculosis

Observation and examination will identify those with abnormal stature, low weight, obesity, Turner's syndrome or hirsutism. In particular, development of the breasts and other secondary sex characteristics indicate the action of oestrogens, provided that there has been no treatment with hormones. Examination should confirm the normality or otherwise of the external genitalia, the vagina and uterus. Investigations appropriate to the likely diagnosis should be pursued including:

1. Karyotype.
2. Measurement of serum gonadotrophin levels.
3. Serum thyroxine and serum prolactin levels.
4. X-ray of skull and pituitary fossa.
5. Examination of the uterus and ovaries by ultrasound.

In those with normal ova menstruation and conception are likely to occur when any endocrine defect had been corrected or in response to one of the ovulation-inducing drugs (see Appendix). In those without ova (demonstrated by high gonadotrophin levels, ultrasound and, if necessary, laparoscopy and ovarian biopsy) hormone replacement therapy may be indicated to produce development of the secondary characteristics and 'artificial periods' (provided that the uterus is present). Women with dysgenetic (streak) gonads (see Chapter 18, p.196) and a Y chromosome are at risk of developing tumours and should therefore have the streak excised. Those with the testicular feminisation syndrome due to androgen resistance or 5 α-reductase deficiency should have the gonads (testes) removed for the same reason, and should continue to live as females in accordance with their appearance and rearing.

Secondary amenorrhoea

This is a symptom which may indicate serious illness, psychological disturbance or a physiological event such as pregnancy. Secondary amenorrhoea, defined as 6 months without a period (excluding pregnancy), affects more than 1 per cent of women during their reproductive years. To many women, and their relatives, amenorrhea is worrying and causes anxiety about future fertility. The fact that menstruation has occurred limits the possible diagnoses and the history and examination will often indicate the cause. Amenorrhoea while taking the contraceptive pill is an unrelated problem, being failure to have withdrawal bleeds, but those with prolonged amenorrhoea after stopping the pill should be investigated in the same way as others. It is important to discover if there has been any related stress (bereavement, disruption of a relationship, travel, examinations, etc.) or marked change in weight. In particular pregnancy, anorexia nervosa and bulaemia should be excluded as far as possible.

Examination should include observation of the weight and nutritional state, the breasts for galactorrhoea, and vaginal or rectal assessment of the pelvis.

Investigations:

1. Serum gonadotrophins
   (a) High levels indicate ovarian failure or pregnancy
   (b) Low levels suggest a pituitary or CNS cause

(c) High LH:FSH ratio suggests polycystic ovarian disease

2. Serum prolactin (raised with drugs such as phenothiazines, hypothyroidism or prolactinoma).

3. Thyroid function tests.

4. Lateral X-ray of skull.

5. Ultrasonic examination of the ovaries (for evidence of ovarian activity, polycystic disease ultrasound of ovary or tumour).

6. Ultrasonic examination of the uterus (the uterus will be a normal size if there is a significant amount of oestrogen being produced and small if levels are basal).

Oestrogen production can also be assessed by measurement in saliva, blood or urine. Repeated measurements, at weekly intervals, will reveal whether levels are constant or fluctuating. The exhibition of a progestogen (e.g. medroxyprogesterone acetate 10 mg daily for 5 days) will usually be followed by a withdrawal bleed if there is significant oestrogen production. It is not necessary to carry out all these investigations and skilled ultrasound examination can give the necessary information about oestrogen status.

Approximately 20 per cent of patients will have weight-related amenorrhoea and another 20 per cent hyperprolactinaemia, but the largest group have no detectable pathology and the amenorrhoea is either due to stress or unexplained failure of gonadotrophin release. Appropriate treatment may be psychiatric, dietary or pharmacological (e.g. bromocryptine), according to the cause. Induction of ovulation (see Appendix) is indicated for those who wish to become pregnant and in whom no other treatment is likely to restore normal menstruation. In those with ovarian failure hormone replacement therapy may be advised. Women in whom an emotional basis is diagnosed, or in whom no specific cause has been found, may be best left untreated since menstruation may return spontaneously. Amenorrhoea is no guarantee against pregnancy and patients should be advised to use contraception where appropriate. Where there is evidence of continuing unopposed oestrogen action or prolonged amenorrhoea, oestrogen and/or progesterone treatment may be given as replacement therapy.

Menorrhagia

Menorrhagia means excessive menstrual bleeding, which may occur as clots or 'flooding'. The woman may notice that her periods have become heavier, which may be embarrassing or inconveniently heavy, interfere with her normal activities, or they may cause anaemia. Fibroids, adenomyosis, endometriosis, and pelvic inflammatory (see p.176) disease may present in this way. It is unusual for malignant disease to do so, but carcinoma of the cervix and of the endometrium can do so. In many cases the heavy bleeding cannot be explained and an endocrine disorder is presumed ('dysfunctional'), though some are associated with anovular cycles. Rarely thyroid or other endocrine disease, coagulation disorders and blood dyscrasias may present with menorrhagia.

Dilatation and curettage (dilatation of the cervix enables the endometrium to be curetted away for histological examination) may be helpful diagnostically. Hormonal therapy with combined or sequential oestrogen and progestogen, or progestogen alone, may control the bleeding. The anaemia must be treated as appropriate. When menorrhagia cannot be controlled in any other way or the patient does not wish to take hormones, hysterectomy may be the best treatment. For emergencies or short term control, amino caproic acid or ethamsylate are helpful. Intrauterine devices cause menorrhagia in some women and this is an indication for their removal; an alternative method of contraception must then be adopted.

Intermenstrual bleeding

Except when bleeding occurs regularly and precisely at the time of ovulation, it is abnormal. It may be a symptom of cervical, endometrial or fallopian tube carcinoma, sarcoma, cervical or endometrial polyps, fibroids, pelvic inflammatory disease, endometritis, foreign body, hormonal dysfunction, cervical erosion, vaginal tumour or inflammation. A careful examination of the vulva, vagina, cervix and pelvis, together with dilatation and curettage is essential to make a diagnosis and exclude serious disease.

Postmenopausal bleeding

This is defined as bleeding more than 6 months after the menopause. The causes are similar to those for intermenstrual bleeding. In this group, however, endogenous hormones play no part unless the bleed proves to be a 'late' period. Oestrogen therapy may be responsible. Rarely there may be an ovarian tumour secreting oestrogens (See Chapter 18). The rule, however, is that after examination carcinoma, particularly of the endometrium, must be excluded by dilatation and curettage. If this is negative and bleeding continues laparotomy and hysterectomy are occasionally required. Atrophic vaginitis usually produces minimal bleeding (spotting) and may be treated with oestrogens if there is no contraindication and other, more serious causes have been excluded.

Postcoital bleeding

This classically occurs as a symptom of carcinoma of the cervix. It may also occur, however, with vaginal pathology, cervical erosions, polyps or endometrial carcinoma. If the cervix is abnormal biopsy is mandatory; if there is no satisfactory explanation on examination dilatation and curettage must be performed.

Polymenorrhoea

Frequent periods, which patients may confuse with intermenstrual bleeding. Short cycles do occur and are often anovular. It is safest to perform a diagnostic dilatation and curettage if there is any doubt about the nature of the bleeding. The cycle may be controlled by giving a progestogen during the whole or second part of the cycle, or by suppressing gonadotrophin and ovarian activity altogether with a combined oestrogen-progestogen preparation (see Appendix).

Table 16.2 Endometrial hyperplasia.

Aetiology: Unopposed oestrogen action
Assessment Diagnosis: Histology for endometrial tissue
Treatment: No typical features — Stimulate ovulation
        or
        Administer cyclical progestogen
        or
        Suppress ovarian activity with combined contraceptive pill
        or
        Danazol
        or
        Hysterectomy

Atypical features — Discuss with pathologist — If mild, progestrogen therapy, caution, regression must be confirmed by regular endometrial biopsy otherwise the safest course is Hysterectomy
If severe, Hysterectomy

Irregular vaginal bleeding

Sometimes described as metrorrhagia. The term is not very helpful and it is best to describe the bleeding, its duration, the amount, and the variation and length of cycle. There is again the problem of distinguishing between periods and abnormal bleeding. Irregular periods are normal for some women, but they are frequently anovular and may occur in association with systemic disease such as diabetes and thyroid dysfunction. Anovular cycles are commonest after the menarche and before the menopause. Metropathia haemorrhagica is a condition in which continued oestrogen secretion leads to cystic hyperplasia of the endometrium and after a period of amenorrhoea breakthrough bleeding occurs which may continue for some time. In polycystic ovarian disease persistence of multiple ovarian follicles is associated with a raised LH:FSH ratio and an increased output of androstenedione and testosterone. These patients, who may be obese and hirsute, can develop endometrial hyperplasia (Table 16.2) and are at increased risk of endometrial carcinoma if the condition persists. Irregular bleeding may also occur in association with stress or emotional disturbance other systemic illness or malnutrition.

It is also important to establish a diagnosis, which requires assessment of the woman's general medical state, endocrinological investigation and dilatation and curettage. An endocrine diagnosis alone is inadequate since neoplastic disease may coexist, and unopposed oestrogen acting on the endometrium predisposes to carcinoma.

Oligomenorrhoea

This is the term used to describe infrequent periods, that is cycles of longer than 6 weeks. The causes include anovular cycles, polycystic ovarian disease and general endocrine disease; alternatively the prolonged cycle may simply be normal for that individual.

In those with anovular cycles, ovulation may be induced if pregnancy is desired, otherwise progestogens during the second half of the cycle (see Appendix), or combined oestrogen-progestogen therapy are appropriate. Thyroid and other disorders should be treated appropriately, whereupon the cycle should revert to normal.

Premenstrual tension

This is a condition which occurs for a variable number of days before the onset of menstruation. The symptoms vary in intensity and affect a small population of women, perhaps 5 per cent, severely. They include nervous tension, irritability, depression, a bloated feeling, particularly of the breast and abdomen, swelling of the extremities and headaches. During this time the need for sleep, allergic reactions and the risk of accident, crime, confrontation and loss of control are increased. The symptoms should disappear with the onset of menstruation.

The cause is not fully understood but hyperaldosteronism, secondary to increased progesterone, may be responsible for the fluid retention or redistribution. It is important to differentiate the syndrome from dysmenorrhoea, and to assess it in relation to the woman's commitments, symptoms and disability. Many of those who suffer severe symptoms are under stress at home or at work, or in both places, and the social stress and premenstrual tension undoubtedly exacerbate each other. Prolonged diuretic therapy may increase fluid retention but spironolactone can be used cyclically when the discomfort is maximal. Pyridoxine (vitamin B6) has been used and in normal therapeutic doses has no adverse effects, although the benefits claimed have not been proved. Progesterone and its stereoisomer dydrogesterone have been given during the second half of the cycle and benefit some women; the oestrogen-progestogen contraceptive pill is an alternative though some women have similar symptoms while taking it.

Dysmenorrhoea

Discomfort normally accompanies menstruation after ovulation. When it is disabling, or interferes with normal activities, and is not controlled by mild analgesics, it is a symptom for which women seek diagnosis and treatment. Primary dysmenorrhoea starts in adolescence, and may increase in severity between menarche and the early 20s. There may be colicky pain or aching in the abdomen with backache and radiation to the thighs. It is thought to be caused by prostaglandins and therefore preparations such as mefenamic acid, flufenamic acid and naproxen are usually effective. Ovulation suppression with the combined contraceptive pill is also helpful.

Secondary dysmenorrhoea is associated with pelvic inflammatory disease, adenomyosis, endometriosis and sometimes with sexual and emotional difficulties. Underlying organic disease must be excluded, if necessary by laparoscopy and, if present, treated appropriately.

Further reading

Dewhurst, Sir John (1980). *Practical Pediatric and Adolescent Gynaecology*. Dekker, New York.

Vanderbrouke, J.P., Van Laar, A. and Valkenburg, H.A. (1982). Synergy Between Thinness and Intensive Sports Activity in Delaying Menarche. *British Medical Journal* ii, 1907–8.

17

Pelvic infection, vaginal discharge

Vulvitis

The vulva may itch or be sore as a result of infection or inflammation depending on the agent and its severity. There are so many possible causes that it is best to group them as follows:

1. Chemical and local irritants or allergens; antiseptics, deodorants, soaps talc, nylon tights, and occasionally contraceptives.
2. Poor hygiene.
3. General or systemic disease; diabetes mellitus, hepatitis, Hodgkins' disease, leukaemia, uraemia, varicella, psoriasis.
4. Sexually transmitted diseases; chancroid, granuloma inguinal lymphogranuloma; herpes simplex, syphilis, gonorrhoea trichomoniasis, condyloma acuminata (warts due to papilloma virus).
5. Other infections and parasites; furuncles, scabies, lice, threadworms candidiasis.
6. Oestrogen deficiency; atrophy.
7. Dystrophies and tumours (see chapter 18, p. 179); note that carcinom and other lesions of this group frequently present with pruritus vulvae

Any discharge from the vagina may cause irritation of the vulva. In young children pruritus is usually due to candida, or threadworms. In post menopausal women the vulval skin atrophies and is more susceptible t infection; it responds well to local or systemic treatment with oestrogen.

Diagnosis

The cause of pruritus or inflammation requires a careful history an examination often with microbiological and other investigations. The cultur of some organisms and the diagnosis of some of the local diseases are difficul The consequences of failure to diagnose diseases such as diabetes or carcinom of the vulva are serious. For this reason it is wise always to test the urine fc sugar, and, where the diagnosis is difficult, to consider the value of a bloo count and biopsy. The vulva can be involved in Crohn's disease and nor specific ulcers may occur on their own or associated with buccal ulcers an iritis (Behçet's syndrome). Most infections involve the vagina and vulv (vulvo-vaginitis) and are described under vaginitis.

Bartholin's gland

Blockage of the duct causes the formation of a cyst, usually 4–5 cm in diameter, which is situated deep to the posterior end of the labium minus (Fig. 17.1). It can be treated by excision or marsupialization (excision of part of the wall, after which the wall is stitched to the skin leaving an opening). If the gland is infected an extremely painful abscess will occur. The treatment is emergency admission to hospital and marsupialization (there is often recurrence after drainage and antibiotics act too slowly). Some abscesses are due to gonorrhoea and a swab should be sent for appropriate culture.

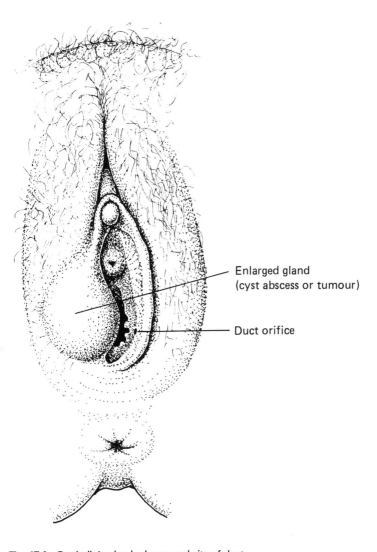

Enlarged gland
(cyst abscess or tumour)

Duct orifice

Fig. 17.1 Bartholin's gland, abcess and site of duct.

Vaginitis

There is normally some discharge composed of desquamated cells, and secretions from the glands of the lower genital tract. Patients may complain of discharge because of its quantity, an offensive smell or associated pruritus. Sometimes the discharge appears abnormal but the patient has not noticed it. The vagina is normally acid (pH 4) and therefore resistant to infection. Discharge from the uterus or cervix, low oestrogen levels, foreign bodies and the use of douches can all interfere with this barrier.

Symptoms of vaginitis

These include discharge, pruritus, soreness and dyspareunia. Ulcers may be due to syphilis, chancroid, carcinoma or trauma. Discharge may come from above the vagina and be due to cervical erosion, cervical or uterine polyps, cervicitis, carcinoma of the cervix, endometrium or fallopian tube.

Causes of Vaginitis

Vaginitis or vaginal discharge may be caused by:

1. Chemical and local irritants or allergens; douches, deodorants spermicides, sheaths, diaphragms, soaps.
2. Foreign bodies; retained tampons, pessaries, sex aids, 'oddities'.
3. Atrophy; postmenopausal with infection.
4. Infection; Trichomonal vaginitis, candidiasis, gonorrhoea, gardnerella vaginalis.
4. Parasites; threadworms.
5. Fistulae; from the urinary tract or bowel.
6. Carcinoma of the cervix or vagina.

A careful examination should enable chemical and allergic causes, atrophy, foreign bodies and fistulae to be identified. If vaginitis is severe, bleeding may occur particularly with atrophy. Removal of foreign bodies is usually followed by a rapid return of the vagina to normal and provided there has been no trauma no antibiotics are required.

Vaginal candidiasis
This is particularly common during pregnancy, in diabetic women and those taking antibiotics. Itching is the usual symptom but there may be soreness and the discharge, which is not generally profuse, may be a thick cheesy membrane (adherent to the vagina) or watery. The vagina and vulva may be red with excoriation of the latter.

Trichomonal vaginitis
This is due to a flagellate protozoon (see Fig. 17.2) transmitted by sexual intercourse. It characteristically produces a frothy greenish yellow discharge with an unpleasant smell and pruritus or soreness, but it can be asymptomatic.

Gardnerella vaginalis
A Gram-negative bacillus producing a grey discharge with a characteristically fishy odour.

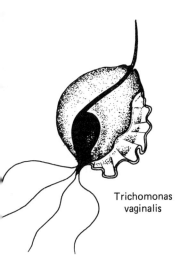

Trichomonas
vaginalis

Fig. 17.2 *Trichomonas vaginalis.* (With kind permission from Sir Stanley Clayton, reproduced from *Gynaecology by Ten Teachers* 14t edn. in press).

Gonorrhoea

This does not cause vaginitis during the reproductive period of life though it can do so in young girls. It may, however, be associated with another infection such as trichomonal vaginitis. Symptoms may include dysuria, frequency, discharge or may be absent altogether. Many cases are diagnosed through contact tracing.

Investigations

Swabs taken from the upper part of the vagina, the cervix and urethra are required for diagnosis of gonorrhoea which is difficult. A transport medium, such as Stuart's, is required if swabs are not plated out immediately. Trichomonads on vaginal swabs will multiply in special media such as Feinberg–Whittington but can also be identified by microscopy if discharge is added to a drop of saline on a slide. A cervical smear may enable the cytologist to identify Trichomonas and Candida. With Gardnerella the vaginal pH is greater than 5.5 and characteristic 'clue-cells' are seen if the discharge is examined in saline.

Treatment

This should include the partner, if trichomonal vaginitis, gonorrhoea or possibly Gardnerella is identified. Coitus should be avoided during treatment.

Metronidazole 200 mg thrice daily for 7 days is used for trichomonal vaginitis. It is also used to treat Gardnerella, dosage 400 mg tds for 7 days. Alcohol must not be taken while on treatment with metronidazole.

Candidiasis
The usual treatment is nystatin pessaries (2 at night for 2 weeks) and the application of nystatin cream. Gentian violet 1 per cent solution applied locally relieves severe symptoms quickly. Other recent preparations appear to be effective in shorter courses including clotrimazole and econazole (3 day course), and miconazole (7 days).

Gonorrhoea
Procaine penicillin 4.8 million units by injection after probenecid 1 g by mouth, ampicillin or cefuroxine may be used, or, if the strain is penicillin resistant, or the patient is allergic to it, tetracycline may be used.

Pelvic inflammatory disease

This term is used to cover infection or inflammation which usually starts in the fallopian tubes (salpingitis)or endometrium, and involves other pelvic organs and peritoneum to a variable degree. Most cases are infective and occur as a result of:

1. Blood borne infection (rare — tuberculosis).
2. Septic abortion (criminal or therapeutic).
3. Puerperal infection (previously common, now rare).
4. Ascending infection, usually venereal (Gonorrhoea or Chlamydia), but can be associated with intrauterine contraceptive devices.
5. Vaginal surgery; hysterosalpingography, termination of pregnancy, curettage.
6. Transperitoneal; appendicitis or abdominal surgery.

Inflammation without infection is most commonly the result of pelvic surgery, haemorrhage or endometriosis. Organisms responsible include a variety of anaerobic bacteria. *N. gonorrhoeae, M. tuberculosis, E. coli, Streptococci, S. aureus.* About 40 per cent of cases are now thought to be due to *Chlamydia trachomatis.* There are many other rare forms of infection and inflammation such as sarcoid and schistosomiasis. Intrauterine contraceptive devices seem to be associated with an increased risk of pelvic inflammatory disease, particularly in young nulliparous patients.

The disease may be acute, subacute or chronic and varies greatly in severity. It may be asymptomatic and, particularly if neglected, can lead to abscess formation or tubal damage, with subsequent infertility or increased risk of ectopic pregnancy.

Symptoms

The commonest is lower abdominal pain, usually bilateral, though it may be more severe on one side. The patient may notice fever, discharge, dyspareunia and headache. Abnormal uterine bleeding is common and the onset or exacerbations frequently coincide with a period. The pyrexia varies according to the severity of the attack.

Examination

There is usually abdominal tenderness with signs which are occasionally gross, for example, widespread guarding and rebound tenderness. On pelvic examination there may be discharge, movement of the cervix may produce pain, and the uterus and adnexa are tender, sometimes acutely so. If there is a pyosalpinx or tubovarian abscess a tender mass may be felt in the fornix.

Differential diagnosis

This can include appendicitis, ectopic pregnancy, complications of ovarian cysts, and abortion. Gastrointestinal symptoms are uncommon with pelvic inflammation; in most other conditions the signs and symptoms are unilateral.

Investigations

Swabs should be taken for culture (including *N. gonorrhoeae*); a total and differential white cell count and erythrocyte sedimentation rate are often helpful. Serological tests for syphilis may be indicated. A plain X-ray of the abdomen is not usually helpful and should be avoided in young women if possible. An ultrasound scan of the pelvis is helpful if there is a mass, lost IUCD or doubt about an ectopic pregnancy. If the diagnosis is in doubt, however, laparoscopy is the best means of establishing it and also enables swabs to be taken from the pelvis.

Treatment

For the acute form this consists of rest (in hospital if severe or the diagnosis is doubtful), analgesics and antibiotics, a suitable regime being metronidazole 400 mg tds for one week and tetracycline 500 mg qid for a week or longer. Signs and symptoms should improve within 48 hours. If there is an IUCD this should be removed. After one attack there is an increased risk of further episodes and the patient should be warned of this and advised to take life gently for several months (i.e. not get overtired, lead a hectic social or sexual life).

Recurrent acute or chronic disease may lead to pelvic damage, continuing pain and ill health. Sometimes longer periods of rest and antibiotics will control this. Pain may take some time to resolve particularly when there is guilt or particular anxiety. For severe or chronic disease which does not respond to conservative treatment surgery may be required, involving removal of the tubes alone or with the uterus and occasionally the ovaries. Surgery in the presence of acute inflammation can be very difficult and should be avoided if possible. A pyosalpinx or tubovarian abscess should be treated conservatively initially, and drained if it does not respond. Hydrosalpinges occur after treated or resolved infection when the fimbrial end of the tube is blocked; they cause infertility and sometimes pelvic discomfort or dyspareunia. (For the treatment of septic abortion see p. 96).

Tuberculous pelvic inflammatory disease is diagnosed from swabs, histology or culture of premenstrual endometrium. It tends to damage the tubes severely and lead to infertility. The primary treatment is with three drugs, usually isoniazid, rifampicin and ethambutol (or streptomycin). After an appropriate interval this is reduced to isoniazid and one other antituberculous drug for a total of at least 12 months, varying according to the extent and severity of the disease, and subject to drug sensitivities.

Further reading

Adler, M. (1984). *ABC of Sexually Transmitted Diseases*. British Medical Journal, London.

18

Gynaecological tumours and dystrophies

Tumours of the vulva

The vulva is subject to all the tumours which affect skin, although certain other conditions may appear as tumours which have an infective or mechanical aetiology (see Chapters 17 and 19). These include syphilitic ulcers and viral warts (condylomata lata and acuminata), Bartholin's cysts, urethral prolapse, inguinal herniae and hydroceles of the canal of Nuck.

Benign Tumours

These include: sebaceous cysts, inclusion dermoids, lipomas, angiomas and hidradenomas. If they are any size, of doubtful nature, or causing symptoms they should be excised.

Vulval intraepithelial neoplasia (VIN)
These lesions are graded I–III. They are being seen more frequently and may present with pruritis, ulceration or an atypical appearance of skin. The only way to ensure the diagnosis, or establish the cause, is to biopsy any area which is irritating or abnormal, or better, examine it with the colposcope. Preinvasive disease can be treated by excision, destruction with the laser or topical 5-fluouracil (this is an extended and painful form of treatment).

Malignant tumours

Squamous carcinoma of the vulva represents about 4 per cent of primary malignant disease of the genital tract. It is commonest in older women, but can occur before the menopause. Symptoms may include pruritus, a lump, bleeding, discharge, ulceration and pain. The lesion may be ulcerating or proliferative and the inguinal glands may be enlarged due to infection or metastasis.

Malignant melanoma, basal cell carcinoma and carcinoma of the urethra are rare forms of malignant disease, other tumours such as sarcoma occur very rarely.

The diagnosis of these must first be established by biopsy. The treatment of operable squamous carcinoma is radical vulvectomy (removal of the vulva, inguinal, femoral and sometimes iliac nodes) unless the patient is not fit for this procedure. Inoperable cases can be treated with 5-fluouracil or radiotherapy. The overall 5 year survival is over 50 per cent; it is about 70 per cent for operable cases and 80 per cent for those in whom the glands are free. Further primary tumours may occur subsequently.

Vulval dystrophies

These conditions affect only the vulva as distinct from general dermatoses. They are confusing, particularly because of a lack of agreement over terminology. The symptoms, if any, are pruritus or soreness. The skin may be atrophic, inflamed, white or otherwise abnormal. It is necessary to determine the types of lesion, and this means exclusion of possible infective conditions described in Chapter 17 and, if necessary, biopsy. Atrophic conditions due to lack of oestrogen should be treated with oestrogen. Preinvasive disease and atypical hyperplasia should be treated as described above; the inflammatory lesion, subject to the exclusion of infection, allergy and atypical change, may respond to local steroid therapy. Leukoplakia, a much used term, now only really means white skin and of itself has no particular significance.

Other terms in use include kraurosis (a form of atrophy) and lichen sclerosus et atrophicus (fibrosis and atrophy) in which the skin may appear thin and smooth like paper. Vitiligo means absence of pigmentation; this may be congenital or acquired, and affect the vulva as well as other areas of the body.

Tumours of the vagina

Benign tumours include

1. Dermal inclusion cysts (burial of squamous epithelium at episiotomy or vaginal repair).
2. Gartner's Duct cysts (remnants of the mesonephric duct up to 5 cm diameter, laterally on the anterior vaginal wall).
3. Fibromas, leiomyomas; rare (they can cause urinary retention).
4. Urethral diverticula and cysts of the paraurethral glands (on the lower anterior wall).

Adenosis of the vagina implies the presence of mucus-secreting glands in the vagina. There is an association between this rare condition, clear cell carcinoma and the administration of stilboestrol to the mother during early pregnancy. Skin tags following birth injuries and condyloma acuminata are common. The tumours should be excised, though large cysts can be marsupialized (see p. 173).

Malignant tumours

Primary squamous cell carcinoma, sarcoma and melanoma are very rare. Secondary carcinoma is common and may arise from a primary of the cervix, endometrium, elsewhere, or from choriocarcinoma.

Preinvasive squamous carcinoma and dysplasia occur usually in the upper vagina with similar changes in the cervix. Occasionally there is a 'field' change including cervix, vagina and vulva. It is asymptomatic, does not stain with iodine and can be diagnosed by colposcopy. Treatment is by laser, 5-fluouracil, surgery or irradiation.

Tumours of the urethra

The commonest benign tumour is the caruncle, a granulomatous lesion (polyps may occur) which can cause haematuria, postmenopausal bleeding or be asymptomatic in older women. It is treated by excision or destruction. Primary urethral carcinoma is very rare, but a small prolapse of the urethral mucosa is often confused with a caruncle in the old. Occasionally, more severe urethral prolapse can become congested and strangulate.

Tumours of the cervix

Benign

1. *Polyps* are common and may be multiple and they should be removed. They arise from the ecto or endocervix and may be composed of squamous or columnar cells. The tip may ulcerate and cause discharge or abnormal bleeding, or they may be asymptomatic.

2. *Nabothian follicles* are mucus retention cysts due to squamous epithelium growing over glands in the transitional zone. They are common and asymptomatic, but their hardness can alarm the doctor who feels them on the cervix.

3. *Fibromyomas* occur infrequently in the cervix compared with the body of the uterus (q. v. see p.187.) They can cause acute retention of urine. (Condylomata acuminata are also found on the cervix.)

Malignant

Ninety-five per cent of malignant tumours are squamous cell carcinomas, the remaining 5 per cent being adenocarcinomas, arising from the endocervix. Sarcomas, which can occur in children, are very rare and will not be further described.

Aetiology
Squamous carcinoma appears to be related to coitus; sexual activity starting early and multiple or, particular 'at risk' partners, probably increase the risk significantly.

Herpes virus type 2, wart virus and sperm DNA have all been suggested as the possible agents. The most frequently affected age group is the 40–50s, though increasingly, the disease is being found in women under 35 and can occur even in adolescence and the early 20s. It is associated with lower social and economic status and there are marked racial differences (it is uncommon in Jews), which may be due to patterns of sexual and social behaviour.

Carcinoma of the cervix is usually preceded by dysplasia of the cervix and carcinoma in situ (now described as cervical intraepithelial neoplasia or CIN grade 1–3) when the disease may be diagnosed by cytology, colposcopy and biopsy, and local treatment given successfully.

CIN 1 Mild dysplasia with a high chance of regression (which may justify observation only).

CIN 2 Moderate dysplasia.

CIN 3 Severe dysplasia and carcinoma in situ.

In many cases the progress from early dysplasia to invasive carcinoma is slow, with regression in some cases of dysplasia. We still do not know as much as we should like about the changes; certainly some women seem to progress more rapidly than others from apparent normality to invasive carcinoma.

Cervical cytology

Cells exfoliated from the cervix can be obtained by scraping the cervix with a spatula and making a smear on a glass slide. This must be fixed promptly and the cells examined microscopically (Fig. 18.1).

The objective is to diagnose asymptomatic preinvasive disease (See Chap. 14, p. 144). If women are encouraged to have smears those most at risk seem often to be the least likely to come forward, so that in addition to continuing publicity it is sensible to 'catch' them when they visit a clinic or their general practitioner for other reasons. Cervical smears are also useful in the diagnosis of *Candida albicans, Trichomonas vaginalis,* Herpes and non-specific inflammation or infection. Where there is clinical evidence suggesting carcinoma a biopsy should be taken whatever the smear result. The cytologist can indicate the degree of abnormality of the cells and the likely diagnosis but the diagnosis must be made by the histologist.

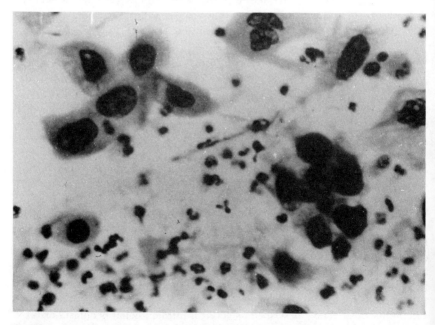

Fig. 18.1 Cervical smear showing dyskaryosis. Note the cells with large dark staining nuclei and mitotic figures.

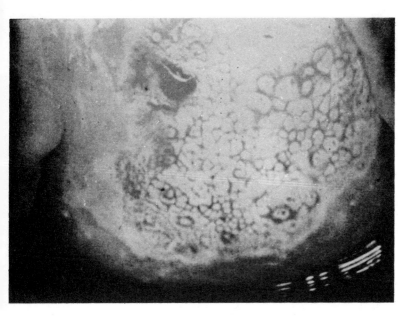

Fig. 18.2   Colposcopy showing intraepithelial neoplasia (mosaicism).

When an abnormal smear is found
The patient should be seen reasonably quickly by a gynaecologist and the likely sequelae explained to her.

The first procedure should always be colposcopy (Fig. 18.2) examination of the cervix using a binocular microscope and subsequent biopsy of abnormal areas identified in this way. Acetic acid is used to clear the mucus, a green filter to show the vessels (which are abnormal in CIN and carcinoma) and Lugol's iodine (which does not stain abnormal squamous epithelium) as a guide to the extent of abnormal epithelium which can occasionally extend into

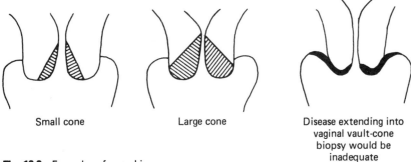

Small cone   Large cone   Disease extending into
                                                  vaginal vault-cone
                                                  biopsy would be
Fig. 18.3   Examples of cone biopsy.   inadequate

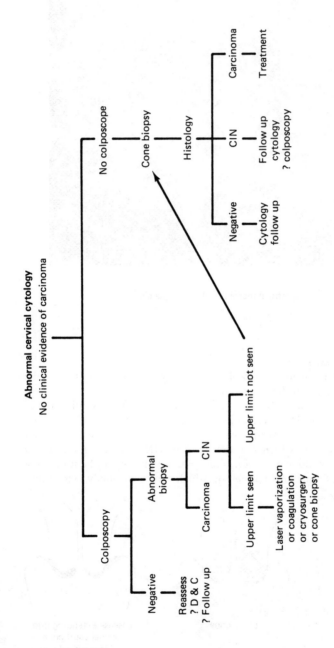

Fig. 18.4 Management of abnormal cervical cytology.

the vagina. It is particularly important to determine whether the upper limit of the abnormal tissue can be seen. If it is CIN can be treated by laser cryocautery or electrocoagulation. In cases where colposcopy is not available, a cone biopsy (Fig. 18.3) is essential to exclude invasive carcinoma and to ensure treatment of the whole abnormal area. The appropriate size of the cone biopsy can be judged best after colposcopy and should not be bigger than necessary since reactionary haemorrhage, secondary haemorrhage, menorrhagia, cervical incompetence and stenosis are occasional complications, particularly with large cone biopsies.

The management is shown in the flow chart Fig. 18.4. Any woman who has had CIN treated should be followed up by cytology three to six months later (with colposcopy if possible) in case treatment has been inadequate or new areas of dysplasia have developed. Occasionally in women with menstrual problems, extensive disease, or those living abroad, hysterectomy may be appropriate (though not generally advised) and cytological follow up is still required. If the lesion extends into the vagina this must be treated.

Carcinoma of the cervix

This may present in the following ways:

1. Asymptomatic (usually from abnormal cytology and subsequent biopsy).
2. Abnormal bleeding; postcoital, intermenstrual, postmenopausal or menorrhagia.
3. Grossly offensive or blood stained discharge.
4. In advanced disease with vesicovaginal or rectovaginal fistula, or pain.

On examination there may be an ulcerating or proliferating tumor, or the cervix may be asymmetrically enlarged. Bleeding often follows examination. With endocervical disease there may be no detectable abnormality and the diagnosis is made at, or after, dilatation and curettage.

Investigation may include a cervical smear, colposcopy and biopsy, which should settle the diagnosis. Urgent admission should follow for assessment under anaesthesia. The extent of the tumour is determined by abdominal, vaginal and rectal examination, cystoscopy and if necessary proctoscopy. A

Table 18.1 Carcinoma of the cervix international (FIGO) staging classification

Stage 0:		Intraepithelial carcinoma (CIN 3)
Stage I:		Confined to the cervix
	Ia:	Microinvasive carcinoma
	Ib:	Other cases
Stage II:		Extending beyond the cervix but not to the pelvic wall or lower $\frac{1}{3}$ of the vagina
	IIa:	No obvious parametrial involvement
	IIb:	Parametrial involvement
Stage III:		Extension to the pelvic wall or lower $\frac{1}{3}$ of the vagina
	IIIa:	No extension to the pelvic wall
	IIIb:	Extension to the pelvic wall
Stage IV:		Spread beyond the pelvis (IVb) or into bladder or rectum (IVa)

biopsy is taken if this has not been done at laparoscopy. Further investigation should include an intravenous pyelogram, blood urea and electrolytes, and perhaps lymphangiography and a CT scan. Table 18. 1 shows the international (FIGO) classification for carcinoma of the cervix; staging being the result of examination, biopsy and appropriate investigations before treatment. Five year survival rates after treatment are shown in Table 18.2.

Table 18.2 Five-year survival after treatment for carcinoma of the cervix (ranges for different centres).

Stage	% Survival at 5 years
I	78–90%
II	43–76
III	20–49
IV	0–12

Treatment
Stage 1a: If the extent of invasion below the basement membrane is less than 3 mm and there is no lymphatic involvement hysterectomy may be adequate. The treatment of this early 'micro-invasive' carcinoma is controversial and depends very much on histological assessment and consultation between pathologist and surgeon. If 1. The depth is greater than 3 mm; 2. there is lymphatic involvement, or 3. a large area of tumour, then radical hysterectomy is probably safest.

Surgery
Generally this is suitable for disease stages I or II, and may follow preliminary radiotherapy. The usual operation is Wertheims' hysterectomy which involves removal of the uterus, tubes, ovaries, parametrial tissue, the upper one-third or two-thirds of vagina, and the iliac and obturator lymph glands. Complications, particularly if the tumour is extensive, include the risk of damage to the ureter or bladder and fistulae; the risk is increased after radiotherapy. Surgery is rarely suitable for stage III or IV, only when the bladder or rectum is involved with otherwise localized disease, or for palliative purposes.

Radiotherapy
This involves local treatment to the cervix and external irradiation to the rest of the pelvis. It avoids the risks of surgery but has its own complications, notably, vaginal stenosis, damage to the bladder (fistulae, irritable bladder or bleeding) and bowel (diarrhoea, haemorrhage, malabsorbtion, fistula).

　　Where there is a choice of treatment the preference and experience of local specialists usually determine the decision. Stages I and II may be treated by surgery or radiotherapy or a combination of the two, while stages III and IV are normally treated by radiotherapy. Adenocarcinoma is preferably treated by surgery as it is relatively resistant to radiotherapy.

Tumours of the body of the uterus

Benign tumours

Endometrial polyps
These are common, vary in size and may be multiple. The presenting symptom is abnormal bleeding or discharge, particularly if the polyp reaches, or protrudes through, the cervix and becomes ulcerated; many small polyps, however, are asymptomatic.

Fibroids (leiomyomas)
These occur in approximately 25 per cent of women over 40, and are particularly common in Africans. They may be single, but are usually multiple, increase in frequency with age and regress after the menopause. They may grow considerably during pregnancy but regress afterwards.

Fibroids are described according to their position in the uterus (See Fig. 18.5). Subserous fibroids generally cause the least symptoms unless they grow large, when they may cause pressure on the bowel or bladder, abdominal discomfort or distension, or may actually be felt by the patient.

Intramural fibroids enlarge the uterus and may be associated with menorrhagia, but it is submucous fibroids which cause trouble most frequently. They may cause menorrhagia, intermenstrual bleeding and discharge. Dysmenorrhoea and particularly severe menorrhagia may occur as the submucous fibroids develop into polyps. Such polyps may reach the cervix where they can be felt; often bleeding on examination or coitus.

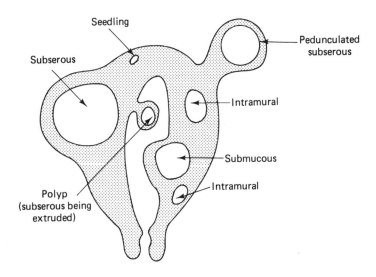

Fig. 18.5   Uterine fibroids.

Complications
1. Torsion of a pedunculated subserous fibroid can occur, though rare.
2. Cystic degeneration — due to the cystic state of the fibroid, it may be mistaken for an ovarian cyst on examination by ultrasound.
3. Calcification is often seen in the elderly; the fibroid may feel rock hard, and shows up well on a plain X-ray.
4. Red degeneration may be due to local ischaemia, this causes severe pain and tenderness with considerable systemic upset including pyrexia. It is most often seen in pregnancy but can occur in the non-pregnant woman.
5. Sarcomatous change in a fibroid is very uncommon. If a fibroid grows rapidly in a non-pregnant woman, or at all after the menopause, it may not be a fibroid at all and, surgery may be indicated to establish the diagnosis.

Treatment   Many fibroids cause no problems and require no treatment. Those that are large (usually where the uterus is bigger than a 14 week pregnancy), causing symptoms, or in which the diagnosis is suspect, require removal. In younger women who wish to preserve their fertility and/or keep the uterus myomectomy (removal of one or more fibroids from the uterus) is satisfactory, though it may carry a slightly higher morbidity than hysterectomy, and there is a risk of further fibroids growing. Fibroid polyps can be twisted off (avulsed) after dilatation of the cervix.

Adenomyosis
This is endometriosis involving the myometrium, and is commonest in women over 40. It is associated with menorrhagia, secondary dysmenorrhoea and an enlarged tender uterus. An adenomyoma is a localized tumour, formed by adenomyosis.

Endometrial hyperplasia
Cystic or proliferative hyperplasia, associated with prolonged and unopposed stimulation of the endometrium by oestrogens, this may be associated with infertility and irregular or heavy periods (see p. 169). It may also be caused by oestrogen 'replacement' therapy. The histological picture shows a thickened endometrium with distension of glandular spaces to different sizes. Treatment with cyclical progestogens, stimulation of ovulation, or gonadotrophin suppression will control the dysfunction unless it is due to an oestrogen producing tumour of the ovary.
   Atypical hyperplasia (sometimes called 'adenomatous') is less common. Glandular proliferation with abnormal cells back to back (due to crowding) may justify this diagnosis which is usually made after diagnostic curettage for abnormal bleeding. The condition may coexist with carcinoma or be a precursor of it; the distinction between atypical and proliferative hyperplasia may be difficult, but if there is definite atypical hyperplasia, hysterectomy may be the safest treatment; reversal of atypical hyperplasia with progestogen therapy can be achieved in some cases, but requires meticulous histological assessment and follow-up.

Malignant tumours

Endometrial carcinoma

This disease appears to be increasing in frequency. Seventy-five per cent of cases are diagnosed after the menopause, but it occurs, occasionally, in women in the 20–40 age group. The disease may be associated with oestrogen stimulation from an oestrogen-producing ovarian tumour, exogenous oestrogens or polycystic ovarian disease. It is commonest in obese women and those who are nulliparous or of low parity.

This is an adenocarcinoma. It spreads directly and by implantation, within the cavity of the uterus, into the myometrium, to the endocervix (where it subsequently behaves like a carcinoma of the cervix) and the vagina. It may also spread through the tube to the ovary. Lymphatic spread tends to be late and blood borne spread is rare.

Symptoms include postmenopausal bleeding (the commonest), menorrhagia, intermenstrual bleeding, vaginal discharge and fever (due to pyometra, a condition where the uterine cavity contains an abscess). At diagnostic curettage the profuse friable curettings may indicate the diagnosis. Careful 'fractional' curettage enables the operator to identify the site and extent of the tumour and whether it has invaded the cervix.

Any patient with involvement of the cervix should be treated as for adenocarcinoma of the cervix (see p. 186); total hysterectomy and bilateral salpingo-oöphorectomy is the basis of treatment for other patients. In cases where the myometrium is invaded deeply, pelvic lymphadenectomy, as in Wertheim's hysterectomy, may be advised. Radiotherapy may be given to the endometrium before surgery, or to the vaginal vault after hysterectomy, but its place is rather controversial as this is not a very radiosensitive tumour. Irradiation may also be used for glands which are known to ∵e invaded, or for advanced cases. Progestogen therapy is effective in producing regression of tumour recurrence or metastasis in 25–35 per cent of cases; usually medroxyprogesterone or 17-hydroxyprogesterone caproate are used. Oestrogens, and progestogens with any oestrogenic effect, are contraindicated. The prognosis after treatment is good, with reported 5-year survival rates of 70–90 per cent, and a reassuring relationship between the extent of the disease and survival.

Tumours of the fallopian tube

Primary tumours of the fallopian tube are uncommon apart from fimbrial cysts which only rarely cause problems. Carcinoma of the fallopian tube is rare and tends to be diagnosed late. The presenting symptoms and signs may be abnormal vaginal bleeding, a profuse pink or blood-stained discharge, and pelvic pain (often bleeding, pain and a mass occur together).

Secondary carcinoma from an ovarian, uterine or colonic primary occurs more frequently.

Tumours of the broad ligament

Fibromyomas, cysts from Wolffian duct remnants and other tumours may occur. In particular fibromyomas may grow into the ligament from the uterus.

Tumours of the ovary

There are nearly 100 different ovarian tumours, many of which occur only rarely. They can be classified according to their histology, aetiology or function. For descriptive purposes they will be divided into neoplastic and non-neoplastic tumours, while endometriosis will be discussed separately.

It is wise to assume that any ovarian mass over 5 cm in diameter is neoplastic until proved otherwise. Clinical and ultrasound assessment of pelvic tumours may be unreliable, because fibroids can be cystic and ovarian tumours solid. Ovarian tumours, particularly malignant ones, may be adherent to the uterus, thus mimicking fibroids.

Non-neoplastic cysts

Cysts occurring between menarche and menopause.

Follicular cysts

These are common and occur as a result of enlargement of Graafian follicles, either as they mature or in the process of atresia. They may be single or multiple and are often found incidentally at laparotomy or laparoscopy. Treatment with human menopausal gonadotrophin, and the polycystic ovary syndrome, are both associated with these cysts. They will often regress spontaneously. Symptoms may occur with the polycystic ovary syndrome (See p. 00) with overstimulation by induction of ovulation or as a result of complications. Larger cysts may cause discomfort or dyspareunia.

Corpus luteum (lutein) cysts)

Usually arise as a result of haemorrhage, which is particularly dangerous in any patient taking anticoagulants. Left alone the blood is absorbed and the cyst will ultimately regress. They may occur in the pregnant or non-pregnant woman. As they are single, the signs and symptoms, if any, are similar to an ectopic pregnancy, particularly if they rupture (resulting in pain and tenderness on one side of the pelvis and a small tender swelling in one fornix). Theca-lutein cysts are multiple and associated with hydatidiform mole.

Common benign neoplasms

Serous cystadenoma

The commonest epithelial tumour, bilateral in 20 per cent of cases which may be uni- or multilocular.

Mucinous cystadenomas

These contain mucus which may be thick or thin, and are less common and less frequently bilateral than serous tumours. Benign mucinous tumours can rupture and implant on the epithelium (myxoma peritonei), resulting in widespread accumulation of mucinous material and progressive direct spread like a malignant tumour.

Benign cystic teratomas

Often called dermoid cysts, these are mixed solid and cystic tumours derived from germ cells. They usually contain structures derived from all three germ layers. Squamous epithelium, with sweat and sebaceous glands, lines most of the cyst wall. The cyst contains a thick greasy yellow substance, often containing hair. Teeth (which show up on pelvic X-rays), bone, cartilage, thyroid, gastrointestinal mucosa and neural tissue are other components which may be found. About 10 per cent are bilateral. They are heavier than the epithelial tumours and are the commonest ovarian neoplasms women about the age of 20.

Common malignant neoplasms

Serous cystadenocarcinoma is commoner than mucinous carcinoma. Papillary growth is often present and may extend on to the peritoneal surface. There may also be a significant amount of solid tissue. Some tumours of borderline malignancy, while requiring particularly careful histological assessment, have a much better prognosis than the unequivocal carcinoma (a significant proportion occur in women under the age of 30).

Mucinous cystadenocarcinoma
These tumours contain mucus and may have papillae and quite large solid areas. Borderline malignant mucinus tumours also occur, but are less common than the serous variety.

Secondary carcinoma
Up to 10 per cent of patients presenting clinically with malignant ovarian tumours may have secondary carcinoma, the commonest primary sites being the breast and gastrointestinal tract. (At post mortem examination the incidence is even higher.) In most cases both ovaries are involved. Krukenberg tumours are secondary neoplasms showing particular histological features, including the presence of signet ring cells in which the mucus displaces the nucleus to one side. Endometrial carcinoma sometimes metastasizes to the ovary and may rarely present in this way.

Complications of ovarian tumours

Torsion   usually occurs with medium-sized tumours, particularly those that are heavy such as benign cystic teratomas. The ovary and tube twist and eventually the ovary is strangulated. Before strangulation occurs there may be mild or intermittent pain. Once strangulation occurs the pain becomes severe and typically the patient vomits. The twisted mass can be felt abdominally or in the pelvis, it is acutely tender, and there is associated peritonitis. The treatment is laparotomy and unilateral salpingo-oophorectomy unless the woman is post menopausal or there is a definite carcinoma. In view of the frequency of bilateral tumours the other ovary should be inspected carefully.
Haemorrhage   occurs into tumours, and is the means by which corpus luteum cysts are formed. It causes pain and the tumour is acutely tender after the event.
Rupture   of a cyst is not very common but is more likely with malignant tumours, because of their thinner walls. It may follow trauma, examination or

occur during surgery. There is usually haemorrhage into the peritoneal cavity and this will be accompanied by pain, peritonitis and sometimes shock. Mucinous cysts which rupture cause the condition of myxoma peritonei, while rupture of a malignant tumour may disseminate malignant cells. Other complications include retention of urine, obstructed labour and infection.

Symptoms of ovarian tumours

Smaller tumours in the pelvis or abdomen may be asymptomatic. Large tumours may cause the following symptoms.

1. Abdominal distension or a mass which the patient can feel.
2. Epigastric discomfort.
3. Pelvic discomfort.
4. Pressure symptoms; gastro intestinal discomfort, altered bowel habit, distension, frequency of micturition.
5. Stress incontinence, occasionally urine retention.
6. Vaginal bleeding may be due to oestrogen secretion of tumour in the uterus or tube.
7. Endocrine
(a) Androgenic — amenorrhoea, hirsutism, voice change
(b) Oestrogenic — precocious puberty, menorrhagia, menstrual disturbance and post menopausal bleeding.

Malignant tumours may present with malaise, loss of weight, anorexia, nausea, vomiting and symptoms of internal obstruction (Fig. 18.6). Occasionally they also cause thrombophlebitis migrans, and rarely, myopathy.

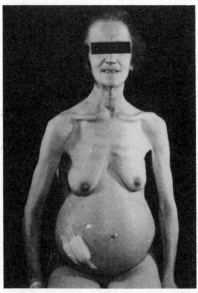

Fig. 18.6 Typical appearance of a patient with advanced carcinoma of the ovary.

Clinical findings with ovarian tumours

The tumour may be felt only on pelvic examination. If it is clearly cystic and on one side its nature may be clear. Tumours may be cystic, solid, or mixed, and mobile or fixed. Their position and consistency may therefore be misleading. A large abdominal mass is easier to assess but it is still impossible to be dogmatic about the nature of most lumps without seeing them, and ovarian neoplasms must be assessed histologically. The presence of ascites, tumour nodules (which may be felt on abdominal or pelvic examination) or hepatomegaly may indicate carcinoma.

Investigations which may prove helpful include cervical cytology (occasionally positive for ovarian carcinoma), chest X-ray, ultrasound scan of the abdomen and pelvis (CT scan if malignant tumour is known or suspected) and radiology of the renal and gastro-intestinal tract when appropriate.

Rarer neoplasms of particular interest or importance

Epithelial tumours
Brenner tumours consist of a fibrous stroma and epithelium. They are solid, usually but not always benign, and may look like fibromas. Endometrioid carcinoma resembles an endometrial tumour and may arise from an area of endometriosis, though it is not often possible to identify this. These tumours may be oestrogen sensitive. Some tumours are undifferentiated and can only be so described.

Germ cell tumours
With the exception of the benign cystic teratoma (See p. 190) these are rare. Dysgerminoma is a rare solid malignant tumour usually affecting only one ovary and seen most frequently in the adolescent or young adult. Endodermal sinus tumour is of interest because it is associated with a raised serum α-fetoprotein level and is particularly malignant. More than one type of these tumours may occur in the same ovary making expert histological assessment essential.

Stromal and special tumours
The fibroma is a relatively rare solid tumour which can grow to a large size. It (like Brenner and other solid tumours) is occasionally associated with Meigs' syndrome in which there are ascites and hydrothorax. If there is a significant presence of theca cells oestrogens may be produced.

Granulosa-theca cell tumours comprise about 1 per cent of all ovarian neoplasms, and are of importance because the cells produce oestrogens. Thecomas, which are rare, look like fibromas and usually behave as benign tumours. Granulosa cell tumours are solid with a characteristic yellow colour; they should be regarded as malignant though they are not as aggressive as ovarian epithelial tumours. These tumours can occur at any age; the oestrogens they produce may therefore cause precocious puberty, disturbance of menstruation or postmenopausal bleeding.

Neoplasms producing androgens are much rarer than those that produce

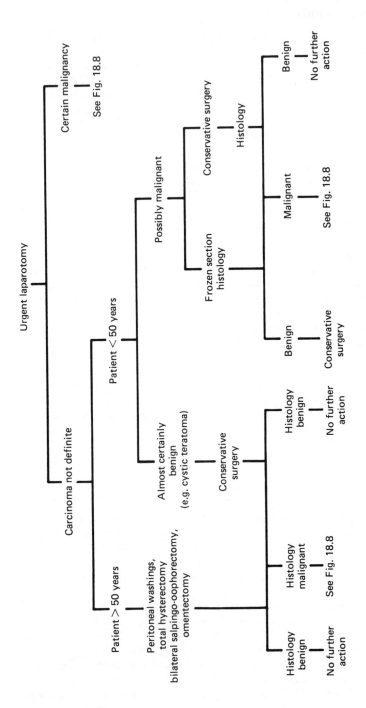

Fig. 18.7 Management of an ovarian neoplasm. Note that conservative surgery implies ovarian cystectomy, unilateral oöphorectomy or salpingo-oöphorectomy.

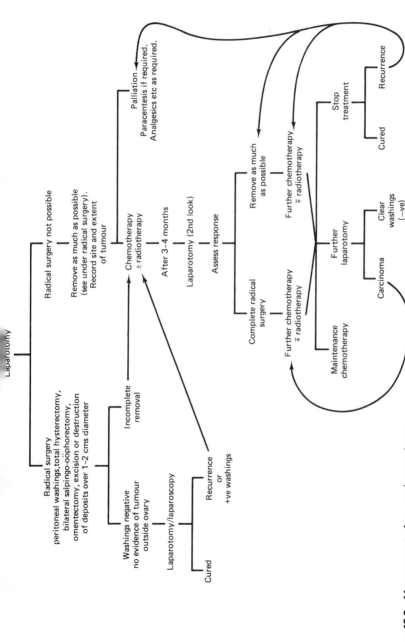

Fig. 18.8 Management of an ovarian carcinoma.

oestrogens and include Sertoli-Leydig and hilus cell tumours; these must be regarded as malignant though cure rates are high. The commonest time for these tumours to occur is in the third decade. The symptoms and signs comprise a loss of feminization, amenorrhoea, hirsutism, clitoral enlargement and deepening of the voice.

In phenotypic women with dysgenetic (streak) ovaries and a Y chromosome or XY mosaicism, there is a particular risk of malignant tumours, notably dysgerminoma and gonadoblastoma.

Treatment of ovarian tumours

The diagnosis of an ovarian tumour usually depends upon laparotomy, removal and histological examination. Once a tumour is suspected, referral, investigation and laparotomy should be undertaken urgently in case there is malignancy. Figs. 18.7 and 18.8 give an outline for management of such tumours.

In younger women it is desirable to be as conservative as possible; tumours which appear benign are therefore treated conservatively, preferably by removal of the tumour and reconstruction of the ovary (ovarian cystectomy). Occasionally there is doubt about the nature of a tumour because of its appearance; sometimes histological reports can be obtained from frozen sections, but the guiding principle is to be conservative unless there is frank malignancy. This means that the histology will occasionally be unexpectedly malignant, and the patient will be advised to have a second more radical operation. In women near or past the menopause it is generally wise to remove the uterus together with both tubes and ovaries, though this policy may be modified to suit the patient's wishes or particular circumstances.

If malignancy is diagnosed clinically, as when there is ascites with a pelvic mass and cachexia, laparotomy should still be undertaken unless the patient is unfit for it. Paracentesis and cytological examination of the ascitic fluid is not indicated since tumour cells may be disseminated, particularly if the tumour is tapped by mistake; a specific diagnosis cannot be made on cytology alone. It is also important to remember that ascites can occur with the benign fibroma and Brenner tumour. Even in advanced disease removal of as much tumour as possible may be beneficial. When laparotomy is undertaken and there appears to be a malignant ovarian tumour the following measures should be taken:

1. Peritoneal washings from the pelvis and paracolic gutters (for cytological examination).
2. Examination of the whole abdominal cavity to assess the degree of spread (palpation of the abdominal and pelvic viscera and inspection of the liver and diaphragm, if necessary with the laparoscope).
3. Total hysterectomy, bilateral salpingo-oophorectomy, removal of the omentum and of any other masses which can be removed. This may occasionally involve resection of bowel. As little tumour bulk as possible should be left, since radiotherapy and chemotherapy are more effective if no tumour mass exceeds 2 cms in diameter

For clinical staging see Table 18.3 (This is based on the operative findings)

Table 18.3 Clinical staging of ovarian carcinoma (based on findings at laparotomy)

Stage I		Tumour limited to the ovaries
	1a:	One ovary affected, no ascites
	(i)	No tumour on the serosal suface, intact capsule
	(ii)	Tumour present on serosal surface and/or capsule ruptured
	1b:	Both ovaries affected, no ascites
	(i)	No tumour on the serosal surface, capsule intact
	(ii)	Tumour on the serosal surface and/or capsule ruptured
	1c:	As above but with ascites or positive peritoneal washings
Stage II		One or both ovaries involved with extension within the pelvis
	IIa	Extension to involve uterus or tube
	b	Extension to other parts of the pelvis
	c	As above with ascites or positive peritoneal washings
Stage III		Tumour involving one or both ovaries, intraperitoneal metastases ouside the pelvis and/or positive pelvic nodes
		Also tumour limited to the pelvis with extension (histologically confirmed) to small gut or omentum
Stage IV		One or both ovaries involved with distant metastases (This includes liver metastases)

The overall 5 year survival rate for ovarian carcinoma is about 30 per cent and the treatment has been intensified in recent years in order to try to improve on this. Surgery may be complemented by chemotherapy and/or radiotherapy and these techniques can improve survival times and the quality of life. The treatment is not pleasant and the side effects of some chemotherapeutic agents such as cyclophosphamide and cis-platinum are not always acceptable. Laparoscopy or laparotomy ('second look'), with the use of modern imaging techniques, enables the result of treatment to be assessed accurately and early recurrences or residual tumour to be treated specifically.

Endometriosis

Ectopic endometrial tissue may be found in the pelvis, particularly in the ovaries, uterosacral and broad ligaments and the peritoneum. It may also occur in the bowel wall, bladder, cervix, vagina, vulva and umbilicus as well as in laparotomy scars. Very rarely, it is present in the thoracic cavity or on a limb. As might be expected it grows under the influence of oestrogen, is not seen before puberty and regresses after the menopause. During pregnancy it is dormant due to the effect of progesterone.

Theories of the origin of endometriosis include:

1. Implantation following retrograde menstrual flow through the fallopian tubes into the peritoneal cavity. Menstrual blood has been observed issuing from the tubes at laparoscopy and laparatomy, and endometriosis is commoner when the vagina is absent or occluded. Implantation appears to be the explanation for endometriosis in scars after operations on the uterus.
2. Metaplasia of coelomic epithelium from which the germinal epithelium and pelvic peritoneum are derived. This would explain the occasional presence of the disease within the thorax.

3. Dissemination through lymphatic vessels.
4. Blood-borne spread.

In areas of endometriosis, endometrium and blood are shed at menstruation and accumulate. The deposits may appear as tiny black spots or larger cysts filled with chocolate-coloured material. There may be local fibrosis and adherence to adjacent viscera, so that a hard mass may be felt. In the ovary large chocolate cysts may be formed.

Clinical presentation

The symptoms often do not relate to the extent of the disease, which may be virtually asymptomatic. Endometriosis may cause secondary dysmenorrhoea, menorrhagia, pelvic pain, dyspareunia and occasionally haematuria or rectal bleeding (if the disease involves bladder or bowel). Endometriosis is often associated with infertility and may be diagnosed during investigation for this complaint; there may be an ovulatory disorder or adhesions.

On examination tender ovarian masses may be felt or there may be an irregular mass comprising the uterus and adherent ovary, bowel or omentum. Hard tender nodules may be felt in the pelvis particularly along the uterosacral ligaments.

Diagnosis requires laparoscopy or laparotomy, and preferably histological confirmation.

Treatment

Small areas of endometriosis which are not causing symptoms may be ignored. Ovarian cysts will require removal to establish the diagnosis. Otherwise the choice of treatment will depend upon the patient's age, her interest in pregnancy and the effects attributable to the endometriosis.

Conservative medical treatment involves suppression of menstruation for a period of 6–9 months, using a progestogen (e.g norethisterone 20–30 mg daily) a suppressor of gonadotrophin secretion (Danazol 200–800 mg daily) or a GnRH agonist. Some patients find the side effects of this treatment unacceptable. There is controversy as to whether medical treatment will cure the disease; it can undoubtedly provide welcome relief of symptoms for the patient and a chance for the reaction to the bleeding to settle (See Appendix).

Surgery may be conservative, involving destruction or removal of deposits, division of adhesions and ovarian cystectomy, or radical. Conservative surgery is indicated where there is a mass, interference with fertility, or symptoms attributable to the disease and not controlled by medical treatment. Radical surgery involves removal of the ovaries and is designed to cure the disease. This should be considered where the family is complete or when other methods have failed and the disease is having an adverse effect on the health and activities of the patient. Since endometriosis is hormone dependent, oöphorectomy or suppression of ovarian activity will arrest the disease. After removal of the ovaries caution should be observed in giving hormone replacement since this may reactivate any residual endometriosis.

Further reading

Coppleson, M., Ed. (1981). *Gynaecological Oncology, Vol 1&2*. Churchill Livingstone, Edinburgh.

Di Saia P.J. Ed. (1983). *Clinics in Obstetrics and Gynaecology — Ovarian Cancer (ch. 10.2)*. W.B Saunders, London.

Fox, H. and Buckley, L.J. (1982). *Pathology for Gynaecologists*. Edward Arnold, London.

19

Prolapse and urinary problems

Utero-vaginal prolapse

Anatomy

The *levator ani* muscles, pass from the lateral pelvic wall to the perineal body, coccyx and sacrum forming the pelvic floor, through which pass the vagina and urethra.

The uterus is supported by the transverse cervical (or cardinal) and the uterosacral ligaments (Fig. 19.1). The pubocervical ligaments may also have some supportive effect but the broad ligaments and the round ligaments have little or none.

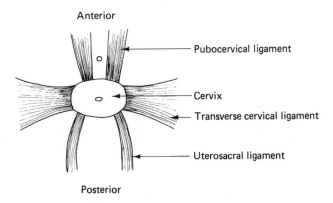

Anterior

Pubocervical ligament

Cervix

Transverse cervical ligament

Uterosacral ligament

Posterior

Fig. 19.1 The supports of the cervix.

The *levatores ani* and the superficial perineal muscles stabilize the vagina, while the bladder and urethra are supported by fascial tissue. The anus and lower rectum are supported anteriorly by the perineal body, while above this, there is only fascia between the middle third of the vagina and the rectum. The fascia and peritoneum of the recto-uterine pouch (Pouch of Douglas) relates

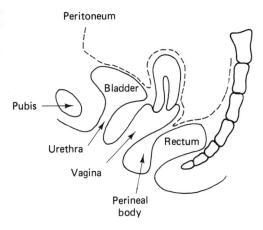

Fig. 19.2 Sagittal view of the pelvis.

to the upper third of the vagina (see Fig. 19.2). Prolapse or descent of any part of the vagina may occur because of the inadequacy of the supporting structures.

Uterine prolapse
This involves descent of the uterus and vaginal vault. In first degree prolapse the cervix does not reach the introitus. In second degree prolapse the cervix descends to or beyond the introitus. In third degree prolapse the whole uterus is below the introitus, often described as procidentia.

After hysterectomy the vaginal vault can prolapse on its own and this is described as 'vault prolapse'.

Anterior vaginal wall prolapse
This allows the bladder in the upper two thirds and the urethra in the lower third to prolapse as well. The terms, *cystocele, urethrocele,* and *cysto-urethrocele* are used according to the area involved.

Posterior vaginal wall prolapse
The upper third of this wall is related to peritoneum in the recto-uterine pouch (Pouch of Douglas) and if there is a weakness a hernia may occur, usually containing bowel or omentum, called an enterocele. The middle third is related to the rectum; a prolapse which includes the rectum is termed a rectocele. This will extend lower if the perineal body is damaged. 'Rectal prolapse' is a separate condition in which the rectum prolapses through the anal sphincter, though it may be associated with vaginal prolapse and rectocele.

Prolapse may be due to pregnancy and delivery, atrophy (due to oestrogen deficiency) or increased intra-abdominal pressure. It is, however, occasionally seen in nulliparous women and in most cases is probably the result of more than one factor, possibly including a congenital weakness of the supporting structures. It is rare in Africans and Indians. The extent to which the conduct of labour can prevent or increase prolapse is controversial, but long difficult labours and the unsatisfactory repair of vaginal tears and episiotomies cannot help. Exercises in the puerperium are designed to restore pelvic floor muscle tone and prevent prolapse.

Symptoms and examination

Prolapse may be asymptomatic or cause the patient only minimal disturbance. (Table 19.1.) Examination should, in particular, include careful assessment of the vaginal walls; often best accomplished in the left lateral position using a Sims speculum and sponge forceps. The patient should be asked to strain and cough to assess the effect. A rectal or combined recto/vaginal examination is often helpful when there is doubt about the diagnosis of an enterocele.

Table 19.1 Symptoms of uterovaginal prolapse.

	Cystocele	Rectocele	Enterocele	Uterine prolapse
Lump protruding from vagina	+	+	+	+
Discomfort, bearing down, heavy feeling	(+)	(+)	+	+
Dyspareunia, loss of sensation	+	+		
Incomplete bladder emptying				
Recurrent cystitis	+			+
Stress incontinence				
Difficulty with defaecation		+		
Discharge or bleeding				+
Backache (so common it is difficult to assess)			+	+

Treatment

In advising for or against treatment, it is important to remember that treatment is only justified if the patient is suffering as a result of her prolapse. Ultimately she must decide whether it troubles her sufficiently to justify the risk and inconvenience of surgery.

Where appropriate, aggravating factors such as excessive weight, chronic cough and constipation should be corrected. In young women it is generally better to avoid repair until childbearing is complete, since further pregnancy may cause recurrence. Physiotherapy is often helpful, but if repair is justified, the patient and gynaecologist must discuss the management of a subsequent pregnancy, the risk and the advisability of caesarean section, or an assisted second stage with an elective episiotomy and repair. In perimenopausal or postmenopausal women, oestrogens may be beneficial. For older patients there is a tendency to avoid surgery but most older women, if properly assessed and prepared, take vaginal surgery well. It is often better to repair the prolapse in an older woman, even if she is not perfectly fit, than to run the risk of her returning later when older, less fit and with worse symptoms which leave the gynaecologist no alternative to surgery. For those, however, who do not want surgery but need treatment, or who are unfit for surgery, ring pessaries are often reasonably satisfactory. These should be changed every 4–6 months and intermittent courses of oestrogens help to prevent atrophic changes, infection, inflammation and discharge. For severe prolapse ring pessaries may be inadequate and other pessaries, such as the shelf pessary may be tried.

Surgery

If surgery is justified the actual operation will depend on the prolapse. Repair of the anterior vaginal wall (*anterior colporrhaphy*) and the posterior wall and perineum (*posterior colpoperineorrhaphy*) suffice for these forms of prolapse. If there is uterine prolapse there is a choice between vaginal hysterectomy with repair, and the Manchester or Fothergill vaginal repair operation, where part of the cervix is amputated and the transverse cervical ligaments shortened. Vaginal hysterectomy is indicated where there is menorrhagia and is preferred by some surgeons in post-menopausal patients. A catheter, preferably suprapubic is usually required after a repair. Complications include retention of urine if there is no catheter, urinary infection, constipation, secondary haemorrhage, adhesions between anterior and posterior suture lines, and dyspareunia or apareunia if the repair is too tight.

Urinary problems

These are particularly common after pelvic surgery.

Urethral diverticulum

Symptoms include frequency, dysuria, discharge and notably dribbling after micturition. A cystic swelling is present low on the anterior vaginal wall and if it communicates with the urethra, pressure causes urine or pus to be discharged. Diverticula should be excised but can recur or be multiple.

The Urethral syndrome

Recurrent attacks of dysuria, often related to coitus and without any evidence of cystitis cause great distress to some women. Single attacks may be due to Chlamydia or gonorrhoea. Recurrent attacks are difficult to explain but may be associated with factors such as allergy to soaps, foams and other substances used locally, the wearing of nylon underwear or tights, lack of hygiene, faecal contamination and coital trauma. A careful history and examination, microbiological investigation and cystoscopy are necessary. If no cause is found, appropriate prophylactic measures may include a good fluid intake, regular emptying of the bladder (particularly after intercourse), adequate lubrication at coitus, avoidance of nylon underclothing and possible allergens, wiping the perineum from the front backwards, and treating atrophic vaginitis with oestrogens. Sometimes the prophylactic use of a sulphonamide after coitus is justified.

Stress incontinence

Urine leaks from the urethra on coughing, sneezing, laughing, jumping or running. Continence in the female is sustained by closure of the urethra; this pressure must be greater than the bladder pressure. The urethral pressure is the result of:

1. Contraction of smooth and striated muscle fibres in and around the urethra,
2. The intra-abdominal pressure transmitted to the part of the urethra within the abdomen,
3. The elasticity of the urethra.

In addition the pelvic floor muscles reinforce the other mechanisms when there is an urge to micturate or a rise in intra-abdominal pressure, and their relaxation precedes normal micturition. If the bladder descends the mechanism of increased intra-abdominal pressure reinforcing urethral closure is missing and incontinence may occur, particularly if there is funnelling of the vesico-urethral junction (the funnelling is greater after vaginal delivery and the menopause). Alternatively a leak may occur because the pelvic floor muscles contract too slowly or inadequately to contribute to the urethral pressure and keep it greater than that of the bladder.

Stress incontinence may or may not be associated with vaginal prolapse. It is important to identify and correct remediable factors such as obesity, and severe cough. Oestrogen therapy may help some women, and physiotherapy (pelvic floor exercises and/or faradism) is often beneficial. There are a number of operations used for stress incontinence, most having a failure rate of at least 20 per cent.

Vaginal repair may be satisfactory for those with prolapse, provided the bladder neck is raised and supported effectively. Although a *colposuspension* (in which the vaginal vault is sutured to the periosteum of the superior pubic rami or the ileo-pectineal ligaments) seems to be more effective for stress incontinence, as it raises the vault and anterior vaginal wall and can be combined with abdominal hysterectomy.

Urge incontinence

This occurs when a woman feels the need to empty her bladder and if she cannot do so quickly leaks or empties her bladder involuntarily. It is usually associated with an unstable bladder which contracts spontaneously. The history should suggest the diagnosis, but in difficult cases cystometry may be helpful. The intra-abdominal bladder and urethral pressure are measured in relation to bladder filling, strains such as coughing, and voiding. Urgency, usually without incontinence, is caused by cystitis, foreign bodies and calculi.

Treatment is often difficult but bladder training, where the patient is taught to empty her bladder regularly but at increasing intervals, and a anticholinergic drugs such as emepronium bromide and hypnosis have also proved helpful in some patients.

Other causes of incontinence

These include retention with overflow, ectopic ureter and fistula. Neurological disorders such as cauda equina lesions, and multiple sclerosis may present as difficulty with micturition or retention.

Fistulae are seen after obstetric, surgical or other trauma, radiotherapy and with carcinoma. Ureterovaginal fistulae, which are usually small, may follow hysterectomy; oral phenazopyridine (100 mg tablet) colours the urine so that identification is easier. Vesicovaginal fistulae may be larger and easier to define. Full investigation including cystoscopy and radiography is required. Expert repair of surgically produced fistulae is usually successful, provided it is carried out after an interval of not less than 3 months.

Further reading

Dewhurst, Sir John, Ed. (1981). *Integrated Obstetrics and Gynaecology for Postgraduates* pp. 631–53. Blackwell Scientific Publications, Oxford.

Howkins, J. and Hudson, C.N. (1983). *Shaw's Textbook of Operative Gynaecology*, pp. 141–86. Churchill Livingstone, Edinburgh.

Stanton, S.L. and Tanagho, E.A. (1980). *Surgery for Female Incontinence.* Springer Verlag, Berlin.

20

Sexual problems

Women with sexual problems may seek help from the gynaecologist. They may complain of a sexual problem or seek a consultation on the basis of another symptom such as vaginal discharge, often taking the opportunity, if the doctor is attentive and sympathetic, to mention their problem or describe it in response to his enquiry. In some cases the patient may seize an opportunity to confide in the doctor during a consultation for some unrelated condition. The patient may mention problems experienced during or after intercourse; notably pain, difficulty and lack of sensation, which may be indicative of pelvic disease or vaginal prolapse. These problems may also be responsible for infertility or arise as a result of the stress of infertility, or its investigation and treatment.

A comprehensive classification and description of sexual dysfunctions will not be attempted here but an outline of sexual function and of the relevant disorders in women and men will be given. The identification, discussion and treatment of these problems requires patience, privacy, time, tact and understanding. Help may be obtained from many sources; interested doctors in general practice, gynaecology, psychiatry and family planning, and from marriage guidance counsellors, psychologists and specially-trained nurses.

The gynaecologist has the great advantage of being able to carry out a pelvic examination when relevant, and should be seen as someone with whom people can talk about their sexuality. Men may also approach the gynaecologist with problems; either with their partner or on their own, or the partner may seek help either on his or her own behalf.

Sexuality and pregnancy

There are considerable changes in pregnancy, with a tendency to decreased sexual appetite, activity and satisfaction on the woman's part, though some experience increased sexuality. There may be an increased inclination to avoid sex, particularly in the first trimester, due to anxiety, vaginal bleeding, previous obstetric mishap, tiredness or malaise. The man may find his partner more, or less sexually attractive than usual and may similarly be influenced by anxiety over the pregnancy. The superior ('missionary') position of the male is best avoided once the uterus is palpable abdominally, and undue vigour and gymnastics are to be discouraged. Recent threatened abortion, multiple pregnancy, antepartum haemorrhage and, of course placenta praevia are relative or absolute contradictions to sexual activity. Sexual activity is usually maximal in the second trimester and decreases again in the third.

After delivery resumption of sexual activity varies greatly. It is influenced by the duration of vaginal bleeding, the general well being of the woman and the amount of disturbance caused by feeding the baby. Sex can play an important part in maintaining and building relationships in a recently enlarged family. A deterrent to the resumption of normal activity is a tender perineal scar after a tear or episiotomy. Patients should be warned about this and the advisability of gentle coitus. The scar should be checked at the post-natal visit and if it is tender or tight it may require revision.

Sexuality after gynaecological operations

In general patients can resume sexual activity when they feel able and interested. Individual surgeons and nurses should give women, and if possible their partners, clear advice about sexual relations after leaving hospital as patients are often too embarrassed to ask. After abdominal operations the woman is unlikely to feel like coitus until her abdominal scar is virtually painless and she is recovering her strength. After major vaginal operations it would clearly be unwise to attempt sex until the vagina has healed and sutures have dissolved; many women prefer, and are often wise, to wait until they have had a postoperative check-up. Again gentleness is required at first if the vaginal size has been reduced (a lubricant such as KY jelly may be helpful). Minor operations need to be followed by only one or two days of abstinence. Some cervical operations, though, (cone biopsy, laser therapy, extensive cauterisation or coagulation and trachellorrhaphy) should be followed by about 14 days abstinence because of sloughing and/or the risk of secondary haemorrhage. The effects of any operation on sexual activity and response should be discussed with the patient before the operation and subsequently.

Assessment of sexual problems

Sexual history

This should include the following information:

The presenting problem   This must be specific (frigidity, loss of interest in sex, etc., are not adequate) with relevant details of the duration and any related factors.

Relevant medical surgical and therapeutic drug history.

Social history   Nature and hours of work, commitment, worry, fatigue level and time away from home. Alcohol intake, smoking, other drugs. Home accommodation. Degree of privacy.

Obstetric history

Gynaecological history

Previous sexual experience and behaviour: Frequency, type/types (masturbation, homosexual, heterosexual, other). Any unpleasant event e.g. rape, assault.

Present sexual behaviour: frequency, appetite, arousal, lubrication, foreplay, time from start to orgasm, orgasm, ejaculation, behaviour after sex, likes and dislikes.

Knowledge of anatomy, reproductive and sexual function

Attitude to sexuality,   nudity, different forms of sexual activity.

Desire for pregnancy or contraception

Religion and beliefs

Childhood experience: general and sexual relationships with members of the family. Any frightening, unpleasant or illicit sexual experience.

Marital/other relationship

Previous advice,   e.g. non-medical, marriage guidance.

Examination

It is important to satisfy oneself and the patient that the genitalia are normal and exclude disease.

Investigations

These may include testing the urine for infection or glycosuria, cervical smear, swabs for culture.

It is important to remember that sexual appetite, frequency of intercourse and sexual performance are particularly affected by factors which the patient may not recognize or describe.

1. Desire for a child.
2. Privacy.
3. Work; worry, hours, fatigue level.
4. Time away from home.
5. Marital relationship.
6. Age.
7. Emotional state; adverse effect of bereavement, anxiety, personal and interpersonal conflicts.

Sexual problems due to disease or injury

Sexual activity may be limited by:

Disease affecting sexual function directly
Conditions such as cord injuries, impaired aortic and iliac artery blood flow, diabetes mellitus, birth injuries ('spastics').

Surgery
A direct effect e.g. abdomino-perineal excision of the rectum renders men impotent; the implications of amputation of the penis or removal of the only testis are obvious. Possible adverse effect on body image e.g. mastectomy, colostomy, ileostomy, prostatectomy, orchidectomy.

Disease or handicaps limiting sexual activity
Respiratory or cardiovascular disorders such as asthma and angina. Musculoskeletal disorders such as osteoarthritis, rheumatoid arthritis and patients who have undergone hip or knee arthrodesis. Blindness which restricts learning about sexuality and sexual experience.

Fear of adverse or dangerous effects on health
This may follow myocardial infarction, cerebrovascular disease, the diagnosis of hypertension or heart disorder, or any other condition which engenders anxiety about physical activity and continuing health. Additionally poor advice from a doctor or too much attention to unsolicited lay advice can render the patient a 'sexual' invalid.

Table 20.1 Drugs which may adversely affect sexual performance.

Drugs taken by addicts
Alcohol in excess or in the chronic alcoholic
*Hypotensive drugs — reduction of libido, impotence, ejaculatory failure
Oestrogens given to the male — loss of libido, impotence
Antigonadotrophins — loss of libido, impotence
Cyproterone acetate (a progestogen with anti-androgenic effect) — loss of libido, impotence
CNS Depressants (barbiturates, benzodiazepines, phenothiazones, etc.) — tend to reduce libido and performance
Cimetidine, Metoclopramide — may reduce or abolish sexual appetite
Any drug causing severe malaise — cytotoxic therapy may reduce libido

*The effects are particularly marked with guanethidine, bethanidine and methyldopa.

Adverse effect of drugs
Taken therapeutically or because of addiction; it may be difficult to discriminate between the effects of the drug and the indication for its use. The genuine alcoholic is likely to suffer reduction of sexual response, particularly impotence. Drugs used therapeutically which may adversely affect sexual performance are listed in Table 20.1.

Embarrassment
The patient may have some abnormality or disease which he/she does not feel able to expose. Examples include asymmetrical breasts, an inverted nipple, hernia, birthmark, psoriasis or other skin disease or genital abnormality (of the pelvis, labia, clitoris, etc.).

Mental handicap or illness
Immaturity, difficulty with relationships or problems in avoiding unwanted pregnancy are some of the many factors.

Management

The aim is to enable individuals and couples to obtain as much emotional and sexual satisfaction as they need and can get. Advice about disorders which affect sexual activity, such as heart disease, should include reassurance and guidance about future sexual behaviour; and physicians and surgeons need to be better informed about sexuality and disease, in order to adopt an appropriate psychotherapeutic approach.

For diseases such as asthma, myocardial ischaemia and painful arthritis drugs such as bronchodilators, coronary artery dilators and analgesics taken shortly before intercourse are helpful. Where there is musculo-skeletal deformity or handicap guidance about coital position may be helpful.

Adverse effects of surgery may be counteracted by measures such as the implantation of a penile prosthesis for the male who can no longer produce an erection, or the creation of an artificial vagina for the woman who has had it removed or was born without one.

The severely handicapped, for example those with spinal injuries, may still have a high libido while erection (and sometimes ejaculation) may be achieved but not felt by about three quarters of affected men. Coitus may be possible, providing complete satisfaction for the unaffected partner and considerable emotional and sexual achievement for the affected man or woman. Touching, massage, masturbation and orogenital sex may be mutually pleasurable or satisfying in addition to coitus or, if it is not possible, instead of it.

Specific problems

Dyspareunia

Difficult or painful intercourse is common and particularly important in gynaecology as it may be a symptom of disease. It may be divided into superficial dyspareunia, relating to discomfort at or near the introitus, and deep dyspareunia.

The causes of superficial dyspareunia include vaginal atrophy, painful perineal scar, muscle tension (vaginismus), vaginitis and dryness. Deep dyspareunia may occur with pelvic inflammatory disease, endometriosis, a prolapsed ovary in the recto-uterine pouch (Pouch of Douglas), hydrosalpinx, ovarian cyst, short vagina, vaginal septum, cyst or stenosis. The treatment being appropriate for the cause.

Apareunia

Failure to achieve penetration; causes include vaginismus and anatomical causes (absence of the vagina, vaginal septum, small introitus etc.).

Unsatisfactory sexual performance

Fears, phobias, ignorance.

Fear or dislike of being touched, hurt or of pregnancy.

Sex Drive   low or very high (not comparable to that of partner).

Poor arousal   Male; difficulty achieving erection. Female; lack of lubrication and interest.

Penetration   Male: failure of erection or penetration. Female; apareunia (failure to be penetrated), or dyspareunia (painful intercourse).

Orgasm   Male; premature ejaculation or ejaculatory failure. Female; orgasm not achieved.

Treatment

It is important to separate patients or couples into groups:
1. Those with specific organic disease or abnormality (many of these present as dyspareunia).
2. Those with psychosexual problems but no evidence of physical disease or of disorder.
3. Those in need of expert psychiatric help. Couples or individuals requiring specialist psychiatric assessment or marriage guidance should be referred to an appropriate expert.

Methods of Treatment

Education
This may involve discussion of anatomy, reproductive and sexual function. Where necessary illustrations and models can be used to help the man or woman to identify and explore his or her own, and their partner's genitalia. The scope of sexual activity, its timing and the proper use or misuse of techniques of arousal may be discussed. Examples of this include per urethral intercourse and brief inadequate foreplay (leading to dyspareunia and/or ejaculation before the woman is significantly aroused).

When two people indulge in joint sexual activity they do what one or both likes and both find acceptable, excluding activities which are dangerous, painful, distasteful or unacceptable to one partner.

The squeeze technique
This is a useful form of treatment for men who ejaculate prematurely. The

man or his partner can practice it, but often the woman does so as part of the sensate focus technique of Masters and Johnson (see below). After masturbation and just before ejaculation (the woman learns from her partner when this is imminent) the thumb is pressed on the frenulum and the index and middle fingers on the dorsum of the penis above the coronal ridge for 3–4 seconds. The degree of arousal, and possibly of erection, is reduced and masturbation can be started again. In this way control of ejaculation is obtained. The next stage of this treatment involves the woman mounting the man who lies on his back. She places her knees either side of his body and leans forward so that she can move her vagina back, inserting his penis. She then stays still while he enjoys the sensation, rising off the penis if he feels near to ejaculation (squeezing may be used if necessary). The penis is replaced in the vagina and the woman starts to move up and down. By stopping and starting they eventually gain control and he can start to thrust. Repeated withdrawals may be followed by voluntary ejaculation, and with repeated sessions control and pleasure increase.

Other useful techniques helpful with disorders of arousal or orgasm.

Relaxation
Muscular relaxation is taught with breathing control and mental relaxation or focussing on some pleasant non-sexual place or object.

Sensate focus technique
The aim of these techniques is to reduce anxiety by concentration on, and development of, other pleasurable experiences (often called 'pleasuring'). It may be used for many disorders, and with other techniques.

Initially intercourse is forbidden, instead activities such as massage and stroking are the focus during the 1–2 hour sessions. The couple are naked together in comfortable private surroundings, and they massage or stroke each other avoiding the genital organs, breast and anus. Bathing, the use of oils or creams, music, and the practice of particular techniques suggested by their adviser may be helpful. The roles are reversed during the session with the active person aiming to give the partner as much satisfaction as possible, therefore communication as to what is pleasant and pleasurable is vital.

Once this stage has been satisfactorily attained (there being no risk of sexual failure), progress to the next stage is permitted, in which the erogenous zones are included but activity is still not intended to achieve great sexual arousal. It may well do so, however, or a further stage may involve increasing sexual arousal to overcome the original problem and lead to coitus and orgasm.

Desensitization
Pictures, film and other visual aids of sexual activity or significance can be used to encourage men and women to discuss sex and sexual problems. The material may include art, humour, pornography or scientific material. By this approach patients should learn about sex, accept their fantasies, improve communication with partners and lose at least some of their anxiety.

Stimulation

This is not entirely separable from desensitization. Men and women are encouraged to seek arousal (using pictures, books, films, etc.), to fantasize, stimulate their partner and communicate more about their sexual feelings and enjoyment. This seems effective for many men, but helps fewer women.

Stimulation by masturbation, however, suggests itself as a means of enabling women who have not reached orgasm, to do so (it is always important however that foreplay should be adequate to lead to orgasm since some men have very little idea of the responsiveness of women). The woman must first learn to know her body, overcome any inhibitions about nudity or touching, and learn to relax. In warmth and privacy she can find the areas of her body where stroking or touching is pleasant or erotic. Then she can attempt masturbation, if helpful with concentration on erotic material. She should always use a lubricant (KY jelly, or baby oil are suitable) and should not expect to reach orgasm immediately. If she does not do so in 20–30 minutes she should stop and repeat the attempt a day or two later. Electric vibrators are occasionally helpful; they can be inserted into the vagina, or more commonly used on the clitoris, or on a finger touching the clitoris.

Surrogate therapy

Selected male or female therapists cooperate with the patient in treatment for sexual disorders and sexual activity. While there is no doubt they can achieve success the ethical position is controversial.

Homosexuality

This is a separate subject and cannot be adequately discussed here. Female homosexuals (Lesbians) generally enjoy their relationships quietly and happily. Recently lesbians have joined the male homosexuals in pleading their case for wider recognition and acceptance.

Males may be homosexual, heterosexual or both. Activities are many, with clubs and organizations catering specially for homosexuals. Sexual satisfaction is obtained in a variety of ways including anal sex, masturbation and orogenital sex. Difficulties arise when homosexuals are promiscuous because of the risk of sexually transmitted disease (and AIDS), and when a wife finds to her shock that her husband is homosexual.

Illegal or abnormal forms of sexual activity

Rape

This is unlawful sexual intercourse with a woman by force or against her will (this can include the use of drugs, alcohol or impersonation). It does not necessarily involve penetration or ejaculation, though if force is used the woman may be physically injured as well as suffering very severe mental trauma. The rape may be by someone she knows, a total stranger or several men. The woman may require medical help to exclude or repair injury, infection and pregnancy (post coital contraception is invaluable in this situation). She will certainly need psychological support and in Great Britain and the United States of America support groups have been formed for rape victims. Any doctor making an examination should do so with great care and sympathy, making meticulous notes. Any injuries, scratches, blood, foreign material or possible semen should be described and samples taken for forensic examination (this is best done by an expert police surgeon if available). Clothing and any other evidence must also be saved. Investigation by the police and a trial are further severe ordeals for any rape victim.

Paedophilia

This involves sexual gratification from children, often by homosexuals. In spite of attempts to alter society's view, this form of sexual activity and its encouragement is both illegal and unacceptable to most people.

Transvestites

Find satisfaction in dressing as the opposite sex. They can be of either sex, though male transvestitism is more common.

Transsexuals

Are those who feel they are of the opposite sex and their role does not fit their phenotypic sex. These people may seek sex change operations, and take hormones appropriate to the opposite sex and behave as homosexuals because of their viewed 'mis-sexing'.

Exhibitionists

Either men or women who find pleasure in indecently exposing their genitals to others. Male exhibitionists, 'flashers', may often masturbate and severely shock their victims, though without any physical assault.

Fetishism

Arousal of sexual desire by unusual sensory stimulation by an object, article of clothing, scent or a part of the anatomy. The obsession with these objects can severely disrupt the sexual and emotional relationships of the individual.

Indecent assault

An offence involving interference with a child or woman, usually touching or attempting to touch the genitalia.

Incest

Intercourse between blood relations, this most often concerns siblings or father and daughter. It is against the law, socially and medically undesirable, but not an infrequent occurrence. Although often concealed, it may be suspected or discovered by professionals (doctors, health visitors, social workers) visiting the home or by school teachers. Skilled psychiatric help is required, usually for the whole family.

Sadism

Sexual pleasure derived from inflicting or watching cruelty (either physical or mental humiliation). This can be dangerous, and can result in severe injury to the partner.

Masochism

The masochist is a person who gets sexual satisfaction from his/her own pain and humiliation.

Further Reading

Masters, W.H. and Johnson, V.E. (1966). *Human Sexual Response*. Churchill Livingstone, Edinburgh.
Masters, W.H. and Johnson, V.E. (1970). *Human Sexual Inadequacy*. Churchill Livingstone.
Trimmer, E. (1978). *Basic Sexual Medicine*. Heinemann, London.

Appendix I

Gynaecological therapeutics

Menorrhagia

Exclude pathology by pelvic examination, dilatation and curettage, blood clotting screen if necessary. (Ultrasound, hysterography sometimes helpful). The amount of loss may be reduced by:

1. Suppression of ovulation with a combined contraceptive pill preparation (see p. 148).
2. In anovulatory or prolonged cycles by
   Norethisterone 10–15 mg daily from day 12, 16 or 19 to day 26
   Medroxyprogesterone acetate 5–10 mg daily from day 12, 16 or 19–day 26.
   Disturbed liver function is a contraindication. Exacerbation of migraine and epilepsy may occur.
3. Mefenamic acid 250–500 mg thrice daily while required.
   Flufenamic acid 200 mg thrice daily while required.
   These and other anti-inflammatory drugs are contraindicated by allergy, peptic ulceration, inflammatory bowel disease, and active renal or liver disease.
4. Ethamsylate 250–500 mg 4 times a day while required.
   Tranexamic acid 1 g 3–4 times a day while required.
   Tranexamic acid is contraindicated by thromboembolic disease.

Dysmenorrhoea (primary)

Analgesics such as aspirin, paracetamol may be used as required;
Mefenamic acid 250–500 mg thrice daily while required.
Flufenamic acid 200 mg thrice daily while required.
Naproxen 250 mg twice or thrice daily while required.
   These and similar anti-inflammatory drugs are contraindicated by allergy, peptic ulceration, inflammatory bowel disease, active renal or liver disease.
   Suppression of ovulation will normally also suppress dysmenorrhoea and may be achieved by the use of:

1. Cyclical combined oral contraceptive therapy.
2. Progestogen therapy e.g. Norethisterone 5 mg thrice daily from day 5–24..

Endometriosis

Suppression of ovulation and menstruation to relieve symptoms or facilitate surgery:

1. Danazol: 200–800 mg daily in divided doses for 1–9 months.
   Side effects include nausea, rashes and mild androgenic effects (acne, hirsutism, voice changes).
2. Combined oral contraceptive therapy continuously for 3 months (see Chapter 15).
3. Progestogen therapy e.g. Norethisterone. Start 5 mg twice daily, increased to 5 mg thrice daily after two weeks.
   Breakthrough bleeding may occur at this dosage which may then be increased to a daily total of 30–40 mg for up to 9 months. Side effects include weight gain, headache, acne, and general discomfort ('bloating'), changes in libido. (It is mildly androgenic).
4. Medroxyprogesterone acetate (5 mg tablets). Up to 40 mg daily in divided doses. It is less virilizing than Norethisterone.

Suppression of lactation

Bromocriptine (2.5 mg tablets): 2.5 mg on the first day then 2.5 mg twice daily for 2 weeks.

Vaginal infections

Candidiasis

1. Clotrimazole vaginal tablets 100 mg or 200 mg. Dose; 100 mg at night for 6 nights or 200 mg at night for 3 nights.
2. Clotrimazole vaginal cream 1 per cent. Dose; 5 g by applicator twice daily for 3 days or nightly for 6 nights.
3. Miconazole nitrate pessaries 100 mg. Dose; 200 mg at night for 7 nights or 100 mg twice daily for 5 days.
4. Nystatin pessaries 100 000 units. Dose; 2 pessaries at night for 14 days (Cream is also available).
5. Econazole nitrate pessaries 150 mg. Dose; 1 pessary nightly for 3 nights (1 per cent cream also available).
6. Ketoconazole (200 mg tablets) 200 mg twice daily by mouth for 5 days.
7. Gentian violet 1 per cent. The vulva and vagina should be painted. This may be used for quicker relief of severe pruritus and discomfort.

Gardnerella vaginalis

Metronidazole 200 mg thrice daily for a week.
See below for side effects.

Trichomonas vaginalis

Metronidazole: 200 mg tablets. Dose; 1 tablet thrice daily for seven days.
   Side effects: nausea, vomiting. Alcohol should not be taken while being treated with metronidazole.

Chlamydia trachomatis

Tetracycline 250–500 mg four times a day for 7 days.

Gonorrhoea

Procaine penicillin 4.8 million units (or equivalent) or Amoxycillin 3 g after probenecid 1 g orally. Other antibiotics, e.g., tetracycline and cephalexin, should be used if the patient is sensitive to penicillin, or if the strain of Neisseria is penicillin resistant.

Pelvic inflammatory disease (causative organism not known)

A suitable regime initially is:
Metronidazole 200 mg thrice daily for 7 days.
Tetracycline or oxytetracycline 500 mg four times a day for 7 days.

Induction of ovulation

This is only appropriate when the ovaries are known to contain ova, serious disease causing anovulation has been excluded, the patient wishes to be pregnant and her partner appears to be normally fertile.

Clomiphene citrate; start with 50 mg daily for 5 days from the 1st, 2nd or 5th day of the cycle. If the response is unsatisfactory increase the dose to 100 mg. It is occasionally necessary to try a dose of 150 or 200 mg.

Side effects include hot flushes frequently. Less common: nausea, abdominal discomfort, blurred vision, breast tenderness. There is an increased risk of multiple pregnancy (5–10 times the normal). Contraindications, active liver disease, ovarian cysts. Caution should be exercised in treating the women with polycystic ovaries.

Cyclofenyl (100 mg tablets): 400 mg daily for 10 days from the 3rd day of the cycle. The side effects seem to be less than with Clomiphene but flushes do occur occasionally.

Gonadotrophin releasing hormone (GnRh) should only be used in specialist units under expert supervision. It is given in pulsed doses at 90 minute intervals subcutaneously or intravenously using a pump (Dose: usually 15 µg.)

Bromocryptine is used specifically when there is hyperprolactinaemia which has been fully investigated (2.5 mg tablets). Start with 1.25 mg at night after food for 3 days then 2.5 mg daily for 3 days then 2.5 mg twice daily. The dosage must be increased until serum prolactin levels are normal.

Side effects include: nausea, vomiting, headache, dizziness, and change in libido. Although there are no known teratogenic effects it should not be given during pregnancy unless there is potentially dangerous growth of a prolactinoma (in most cases it is discontinued as soon as pregnancy is diagnosed).

Oestrogen deficiency

In women with gonadal dysgenesis, after bilateral oöphorectomy and those with symptoms after the menopause.

Oestrogen therapy is generally contraindicated by a history of breast or endometrial carcinoma, cerebrovascular accident, cardiac or thromboembolic disease. Unless a woman has had a hysterectomy, the oestrogen should be given cyclically with a progestogen during the second half of the cycle. Caution should be exercised if there is liver disease or hypertension.

Vaginal route
Dienoestrol cream (0.025 per cent): 1 vaginal applicatorfull inserted at night for 2 weeks.

Subcutaneous implant
Oestradiol 25–50 mg. Add an oral progestogen (e.g. Medroxyprogesterone acetate 5 mg daily) when appropriate for 14 days out of every 28. Implants will last approximately 3 months.

Oral treatment
Ethinyl Oestradiol 10–20 μg daily continuously, or for 21 days out of every 28. Add an oral progestogen if appropriate.
Combined preparations available include.

1. Prempak C (Ayerst), Conjugated oestrogens 0.625 mg (28 maroon oval tablets) or 1.25 mg (28 yellow oval tablets), Norgestrel 0.15 mg 12 brown tablets); 1 maroon (or yellow tablet) for 16 days then 1 maroon (or yellow) tablet and 1 brown tablet daily for 12 days.
2. Cyclo-Progynova 1 mg (Schering). Oestradiol valerate 1 mg (beige) 11 tablets, oestradiol valerate 1 mg and levonorgestrel 0.25 mg (brown) 10 tablets; 1 beige tablet daily for 11 days followed by 1 brown tablet daily for 10 days and then a 7 day interval.
3. Cyclo-Progynova 2 mg (Schering). Oestradiol valerate 2 mg (white) 11 tablets, oestradiol valerate 2 mg and levonogestrel 0.5 mg (brown) 10 tablets; 1 white tablet for 11 days followed by 1 brown tablet daily for 10 days and then a 7 day interval.

In a patient still menstruating these preparations should be started on the 5th day of the cycle.

Postponing a period

1. This can be achieved for weddings, sporting events, examinations, if due notice is given, by taking a fixed dose combined oral contraceptive for longer than 21 days either to postpone the 'period' until after the event, or to adjust the timing of the cycle ahead of the event.
2. The period can be delayed by taking Norethisterone or medroxyprogesterone 5 mg twice daily starting 2 days before the period is due and continuing until the event is over (bleeding will normally start 48 hours after stopping treatment).
3. Side effects; breakthrough bleeding may occur, particularly if therapy is continued longer than 7 days. The premenstrual discomfort experienced by some women is unacceptable and it is unwise to try this regime for the first time if the event is important e.g., an examination.

Premenstrual tension

No single treatment is generally effective. The following help some women and the choice will depend on the type and severity of symptoms and patient acceptability. Treatment is started to cover the days when symptoms are distressing unless stated otherwise.

1. Progesterone 200–400 mg by suppository or pessary daily (suppositories 200 and 400 mg).
   Progesterone 5–10 mg daily by intramuscular injection.
2. Dydrogesterone 20–40 mg daily from day 12–26 (20 mg tablets) or on the days affected.
3. Spironolactone 25–50 mg daily (25 mg tablets).
4. A combined oral contraceptive given in the normal way (see p. 148).
5. Pridoxine (Vitamin B_6) 100 mg daily.
6. Mefenamic acid 250 mg tds on the days affected.

Appendix II

Therapeutic substances equivalent names in the USA

Bromocryptine	Bromocryptine
Clomiphene citrate	Clomiphene citrate
Clotrimazole	Clotrimazole
Cyclofenyl	———
Danazol	Danazol
Dienoestrol	Dienestrol
Dydrogesterone	Dydrogesterone
Econazole	———
Ethamsylate	———
Ethinyloestradiol	Ethinylestradiol
Flufenamic acid	———
Gonadotrophin releasing hormone or Lutenizing hormone releasing hormone)	Gonadotropin releasing hormone
Ketoconazole	Ketoconazole
Medroxyprogesterone acetate	Medroxyprogesterone acetate
Mefenamic acid	Mefenamic acid.
Metronidazole	Metronidazole
Miconazole nitrate	Miconazole nitrate
Naproxen	Naproxen
Norethisterone	Norethindrone
Nystatin	Nystatin
Oestradiol	Estradiol
Oxytetracycline	Oxytetracycline
Procaine penicillin	Procaine penicillin
Progesterone	Progesterone
Pyridoxine	Pyridoxin
Spironolactone	Spironolactone
Tetracycline	Tetracycline
Tranexamic acid	———

Index